THE
LEUCINE
FACTOR
DIET

THE LEUCINE FACTOR DIET

THE SCIENTIFICALLY PROVEN APPROACH TO COMBAT SUGAR, BURN FAT AND BUILD MUSCLE

DR. VICTOR PRISK

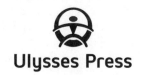

Ulysses Press

Published in the U.S. by
ULYSSES PRESS
P.O. Box 3440
Berkeley, CA 94703
www.ulyssespress.com

ISBN: 978-1-61243-525-1
Library of Congress Control Number: 2015944220

Printed in Canada by Marquis Book Printing

10 9 8 7 6 5 4 3 2 1

Acquisitions Editor: Casie Vogel
Managing Editor: Claire Chun
Project Editor: Renee Rutledge
Editor: Susan Lang
Indexer: Sayre Van Young
Front cover design: Rob Handley
Interior design/layout: what!design @ whatweb.com
Cover photographs: front © VladislavStarozhilov/ThinkstockPhotos.com;
    back © Alex Jones

Distributed by Publishers Group West

NOTE TO READERS: This book has been written and published strictly for informational and educational purposes only. It is not intended to serve as medical advice or to be any form of medical treatment. You should always consult your physician before altering or changing any aspect of your medical treatment and/or undertaking a diet regimen, including the guidelines as described in this book. Do not stop or change any prescription medications without the guidance and advice of your physician. Any use of the information in this book is made on the reader's good judgment after consulting with his or her physician and is the reader's sole responsibility. This book is not intended to diagnose or treat any medical condition and is not a substitute for a physician.

This book is independently authored and published and no sponsorship or endorsement of this book by, and no affiliation with, any trademarked brands or other products mentioned within is claimed or suggested. All trademarks that appear in ingredient lists and elsewhere in this book belong to their respective owners and are used here for informational purposes only. The authors and publishers encourage readers to patronize the quality brands mentioned and pictured in this book.

I dedicate this book to my friends, family, patients, and colleagues who inspire me to continue helping others and effect change in the world one goal at a time.

TABLE OF CONTENTS

INTRODUCTION

Welcome to *The Leucine Factor Diet!* As an orthopedic surgeon with a history of competition in multiple sports and involvement in sports nutrition research, I wrote *The Leucine Factor Diet* to help athletes, performing artists, and everyday people organize their lives with goals and objective measures to overcome procrastination, maximize health, and improve longevity. G.A.I.N., an acronym I live by, explains how you can improve the mind-body connection while fueling both your mind and your body with essential nutrients, dietary supplementation, effective exercise, and medical awareness. G.A.I.N. is an acronym for:

G: Graded exercise—Objectively measure steady progress toward your physical goals.

A: Attitude—Cultivate a positive mental attitude for motivation and recovery from hard work.

I: Integrated medicine—Incorporate proven scientific principles and injury prevention.

N: Nutrition—Attain your performance goals with well-balanced meals and nutritional supplementation.

I wrote *The Leucine Factor Diet* to elaborate on the "N" in G.A.I.N. This book presents an in-depth view of my dietary and supplement recommendations based on health, physique, and performance goals. If your goal is to build muscle, get lean, or just maintain your health, the book will give you the tools you need to succeed.

We are all at risk for injury, disease, and disability. Despite all of our knowledge and experience, our nation is getting sicker—the rates of obesity, diabetes, cancer, and heart disease are rising—and there are more injuries in sport. Despite our desire to blame genetics and the world around us, our health is almost completely in our control. The majority of health issues and injuries are due to lifestyle choices. Whether you eat too much, smoke tobacco, drink alcohol, sit on your butt, or even exercise too much, you are in control of the consequences. Exercise too much? Yes, too much of a good thing can be bad.

This book isn't about low-carb dieting; it's about understanding that your focus should be on the essential nutrients for your health and your goals. *You must eat to live before you can live to eat.* Eating healthy can be enjoyable, but it must include the essentials for good health. We know that there are essential fats and essential components of proteins called amino acids that we can't live without. However, sugars are not essential and can even be deadly to overconsume.

If your goal is to be a superhero with strength and vitality (not to mention a spandex-worthy body), sugar is the kryptonite that can make you weak. It leads to increased fats in the blood and around the belly. It causes inflammation in the blood vessels and throughout the body, leading to joint pain and weakness. It saps the mind and corrupts thoughts like a drug as science clearly shows that sugar is addictive.

Fortunately, nature has provided us with "anti-kryptonite": leucine, a little-known component of protein that is the subject of this book. It turns out that leucine can combat the harmful effects of sugar and make muscles stronger. It improves metabolism and blood pressure. It helps us age with vitality and stronger bodies. Combined with other nutrients from the sun (Superman got his strength from our yellow sun), leucine has even greater power to keep you strong.

This book will help you focus on the essential nutrients in your meals. It will help you optimize the leucine content of those meals. Furthermore, it will teach you to create meal plans that fit your goals. Want to stay healthy, build muscle, get lean, or a combo of the three? *The Leucine Factor Diet* will help you in getting started, in building your plan, and in implementing it. With additional tools and pearls of wisdom, you'll avoid distractions on the road to achieving your goal. It will give you methods to follow your progress, create tasty meals, and adjust to stress along the way. With extra attention to nutrient supplementation and timing, you will get the best results possible.

Enjoy reading this book. Leave comments in the margins on the content most relevant to your situation. Use stickers to flag sections of the book that you'd like to revisit or share with others. If you have questions or just want to continue the leucine conversation, join me on social media @victorprisk on Twitter and Instagram. Follow my blog at LeucineFactor.com.

1

FACT VERSUS MYTH

Understanding how nutrition affects your health, well-being, and leanness is a daunting task. It is so easy to be led in the wrong direction and to put yourself in a worse place than where you started. As an athlete and physician, I never thought that I could be misled about nutrition and lifestyle. Unfortunately, I was naive about the powers of persuasion and the misrepresentation of data.

As a gymnast, I became deeply interested in how nutrition could improve my performance. I frequented the local GNC store looking for protein and supplements to boost my athletic performance. I read magazines like *Muscular Development* and *Muscle & Fitness* for the information they presented on training, nutrition, and medicine. I watched the news, occasionally read articles in newspapers, and surfed the net in its early days.

One of the biggest misconceptions I harbored was that the entirety of my performance developed from hard work inside the gym. I understood that I needed extra protein and vitamins, but I believed the common saying that "pain was weakness leaving the body." Thus, I trained like a beast during every gymnastics practice and weight-training session. I sacrificed rest and sleep to maintain school grades and training. The reality would catch up with me on Santa Monica State Beach in 2005.

I was doing a photo shoot with Bill Comstock for *Iron Man Magazine.* I was on the beach early in the morning preparing for a shoot that would involve gymnastics and partnering skills with my girlfriend. Holding on to my desire to continue with my gymnastics career while working as an orthopedic surgery resident, basically burning the candle at both ends, I approached the rusty metal rings on the beach. You see, for the weeks prior, I had been training with my typical white-hot intensity—working out in the gymnastics gym, hitting the weights pretty hard to become a bodybuilder, and learning to care for fractured bones in the hospital. Little did I know the moments that followed would be a major wake-up call.

I jumped up on the rings to show off a little. I pulled my body into an iron-cross position and held it effortlessly. Then my ego wrote a check my body couldn't cash. I pulled up from the iron cross into a Maltese cross with my legs parallel to the ground. As I did this, we all heard a loud CRACK. Jumping down from the rings with the realization that my bicep tendon had just ruptured from the bone, tears welled up. I knew that I would need surgery. I knew right then and there that my medical, gymnastics, and bodybuilding careers were at a crossroads. I would never do an iron cross again as I couldn't risk another 8-week layoff from the operating room and patient care. Would my bicep ever look the same again? This was a temporarily devastating but eye-opening experience.

After months of recovery and hanging up the gymnastics grips for good, I began to realize that even with all of my medical training and experience in the gym, I was being hindered by myths. Myths that would rob me of my strength and longevity in sport. I believed that fat-free meant guilt-free. I believed that all proteins and calories were created equal. I believed that I was invincible. As you will learn in this book, I was sorely mistaken and the deceptions don't end there.

The Leucine Factor Diet expands upon these myths and gives you the wisdom that I wish I had going into my pursuit of physical performance. I had to learn much of this through pain and disappointment, despite all of my experience and medical training. This book gives you the benefit of all my wisdom from "doing it the hard way."

My twin brother, Tony, was one of the first people to utilize my experience to avoid the mistakes that I made. Tony was always active, but he fell victim to the same myths that we were brought up with and that plague the lifestyles of most Americans. He never paid attention to the quality of his proteins, he ate too few green vegetables, he trained the same body parts over and over without variety, and he didn't take time to recover from stress. In recent years, he came to me saying he wanted to get in shape but was eating children's cereal for breakfast and running only 2 days per week.

Once on the Leucine Factor Diet, he learned the importance of meal planning, resistance exercise to build muscle as metabolic currency (muscle is very metabolically active tissue and is essential to healthy metabolism and caloric expenditure), and techniques to improve recovery. He learned how to find proteins rich in leucine and to eat them at regular intervals five times per day. He learned how to recognize the hidden sugar in foods. He learned how to optimize nutrient timing and how to use nutritional supplements to enhance his energy during the day and in the gym. Now he is leaner, healthier, and stronger than he was in college.

MISGUIDED: CUTTING ESSENTIAL FATS

It is a very painful realization to find out that everything you learned about food and a healthy lifestyle is wrong. Despite all of our technological advances, humans are just not getting healthier or leaner. Current dieting trends have led to increased rates of obesity and the dreaded metabolic syndrome.

Metabolic syndrome is a combination of elevated blood cholesterol and triglycerides, high blood pressure, high blood sugar, and obesity, all of which increase the risk for heart disease and early death. Many of us have been set on this course by false beliefs and misdirection about the foods we eat. This misdirection has come from everywhere. Multimedia dominate our understanding of the world; our TVs, computers, smart phones, and social media are voices for manufacturers, politicians, and government regulatory bodies. Do you believe everything you read, hear, or see? How can you really know what is true?

The trend over the past 35 years has been to restrict calories by cutting fat from our diets. In the 1980s, the fat-free fad was driven by misguided science and government regulation of foods. Accordingly, the food industry replaced palatable vilified fats with even more palatable sugar. This led to an infiltration of high-carbohydrate, low-fat foods into our diets, followed by a metabolic plague of self-perpetuating lifestyle-related ailments like diabetes and cardiovascular disease.

The problem with the concept of low-fat foods comes down to understanding the concept of *essential macronutrients*. "Essential" refers to a nutrient that we can't live without. In other words, our bodies can't make these nutrients from other nutrients that we eat; they must be in our diets. To stay alive and healthy, we must consume essential nutrients like vitamins and minerals.

Macronutrients are the fats, proteins, and carbohydrates that supply calories for energy and building blocks for repairing tissues in our bodies. Of the three macronutrients, two are essential in our diets. The fats we eat are made of essential and nonessential fats. The proteins we eat are made of essential and nonessential amino acids. This leaves carbohydrates as the only nonessential macronutrient. There are no specific carbohydrates that we can't live without (for more information, see Fiber, an Essential Carbohydrate? on page 109). This is because our bodies have the ability to make glucose, the carbohydrate carried in the bloodstream, from the amino acids and fats that we consume.

Thus, you can see how one of the biggest mistakes the food industry could have made 35 years ago was to remove an essential macronutrient, like fats, and replace it with the only nonessential one, carbohydrates. Pulling our attention away from the importance of the essential fats and amino acids has resulted in rapid rises in obesity and lifestyle-related diseases. Belief in a low-fat, high-carbohydrate diet has led to tendencies to store food as fat, to lose muscle, and for decreased longevity.

Another problem is the proliferation of inexpensive processed foods. These come in the form of boxed, bagged, and canned foods in the grocery store. They also come in the form of mystery meats and cardboard buns in fast food restaurants. These foods are heavily advertised, are dirt cheap to make, and have less nutritional value than mud. However, many see a cheeseburger, fries, and a soft drink as a meal fit for daily lunch. Often, the reality is that the nutritional value of any of those quasi-foods has been completely processed out. What you see really isn't what you get.

It nauseates me to realize how long I fell for this marketing. Until I injured my bicep tendon and embarked on the road to bodybuilding success, I would regularly grab lunch at a fast food joint. Food marketing gives us a false sense of what is healthy and nutritious, and we need to educate ourselves and others to avoid being taken advantage of. *The Leucine Factor Diet* will help you to avoid these pitfalls.

THE BLAME-IT-ON-YOUR-GENES MYTH

For the first time in the recorded history of humans, lifestyle diseases like diabetes, heart disease, stroke, and some cancers kill more people than communicable diseases and war. Most of us don't even realize that our misguided lifestyles are creating this problem. Patients often say to me that they are overweight and out of shape because of their genetics. They tell me, "I eat healthy; I just have a slow metabolism." Meanwhile they're holding a 20-ounce regular soft drink and can't tell me what they had for breakfast, lunch, or dinner the day before.

I don't blame patients for this attitude. Many people just don't know any better, and the world around us doesn't make it any easier. Unfortunately, media exposure in the form of advertisements, TV commercials, and the evening news can be incredibly confusing when it comes to nutrition and lifestyle. Newscasts focus on genes as the source of extra belly fat, appetite, and vices. They play the blame game with genes. The teaser might be something like this: "Did you know your genes can make you fat? More at 5." In essence, they turn new scientific discoveries into marketing tools to bring more people to their broadcasts.

The scientific information is twisted to make you feel better. If you are overweight and someone tells you that it's not your fault but rather your genes, that takes the responsibility for your weight off your shoulders. My parents were fat, so I'm doomed to be fat. As I hope you will see or already realize, your daily decision making has much greater influence on your health than your genetics.

In reality, less than a third of our health in general, including susceptibility and performance ability, is really related to our genes. The environment has a much greater impact except in the cases of rare, life-threatening genetic disorders. The studies presented by newspapers and the evening news are being interpreted by one reporter or news agency and may be dictated by agendas or advertising dollars.

The numbers don't lie. When it comes to our greatest health problems, environmental factors can be identified as a cause in up to 90% of those problems. The three most dominant chronic health conditions afflicting Americans (type 2 diabetes, coronary artery disease, and cancers) are largely caused by environmental factors. For instance, smoking leads to lung cancer; eating too much sugar leads to diabetes.

Unequivocal evidence in the scientific literature supports the notion that all environmental factors combined, including physical inactivity, account for the majority of chronic health conditions. A Scandinavian twin study showed that more than 68% of site-specific cancers had a known environmental origin. The Harvard Center for Cancer Prevention estimated that, of the total number of cancer deaths, 30% were due to tobacco, 30% to diet and obesity, 5% to occupational hazards, and 2% to environmental factors.

Low-fiber diets lacking vegetables have been linked to colon cancer.

In a study of 84,000 female nurses, 91% of the cases of type 2 diabetes and 82% of the coronary artery disease cases could be attributed to bad habits and so-called high-risk behavior: being overweight, eating a diet low in fiber and high in unhealthy trans fat, consuming too much sugar, living a sedentary lifestyle, and smoking. Simply put, the majority of deaths from chronic health conditions have an environmental origin. That is, an origin that you can control.

Treating these diseases, and the futile attempts to cure the unhealthy lifestyles behind them, costs a fortune: more than one-seventh of our gross domestic product. That is one-seventh of all the goods and services produced by the United States at any given time. The crazy thing is that the diseases can be prevented by doing things that cost no extra money, mainly making healthy lifestyle changes.

For example, if you have a sedentary job, you will have less non-exercise activity thermogenesis (NEAT). NEAT is the generation of body heat throughout the day and a large portion of your calorie burn. It is important to realize that exercise is not the only way to burn calories. If you sit a lot, you need to take measures to change. This can include changing habits or your environment. In addition to moving more, when you are sitting, you can turn fat burning on by lowering the room temperature (to 65°F), eating protein-rich foods, and using thermogenic supplements like cayenne pepper extract. Remember, you can control your environment and overcome almost any genetic predisposition.

> Thermogenic supplements are those that boost metabolism to enhance fat burning. Pepper extracts are effective in boosting metabolism.

Are there lurking negative effects of sitting idle during the workday? Statistics say yes. Bus drivers and those with sedentary office jobs have nearly twice the rate of cardiovascular disease compared with people who have standing and walking jobs. Research shows that there's a progressive inverse relationship between risk of death from all causes and non-exercise activity in women. Sitting is the new smoking. Does this make you want to buy one of those treadmill desks?

THE OJ CONUNDRUM

Let's take media distractions a step farther. Commercials from our childhood make an indelible impression on our minds that marketers take advantage of. The worst of this comes from the sweetened breakfast cereal commercials we were inundated with as children. Let's be clear from the start: Breakfast cereal with milk doesn't make a complete breakfast even if you add a slice of toast and a glass of orange juice.

A big problem arises in the form of a tall glass of orange juice. Orange juice ads make their juice look like pure energy from the sun ready to fuel your body. But seriously, how much nutrition is in an 8-ounce glass of OJ? Water, sugar, vitamin C, folate, thiamine, antioxidants, and some added nutrients such as calcium and vitamin D. Even though the antioxidant and vitamin content may be of value, if I added these nutrients to a can of regular soda, would you still consider that soda a nutritious part of a "balanced" breakfast? If you read a food label on which the first ingredient is water and the second ingredient sugar, would you find that food nutritious?

To understand the effect that sugars have on metabolism, let's look at the physiology. When you drink a glass of OJ, or sugar water for that matter, the result is a rapid rise in blood sugar levels because the sugar (glucose) from the OJ is rapidly absorbed. It is important for the body to quickly clear high levels of glucose from the blood to avoid damage to tissues. Glucose acts as a toxin to blood vessels, essentially "caramelizing" them, which leads to inflammation and disease.

Insulin is the hormone responsible for getting sugar out of the blood and putting it into tissues like the liver, fat, and muscle. Once you drink rapidly absorbed sugar water, insulin is released just as quickly to clear it from the blood. It is important to realize that insulin isn't bad; the fact that it clears toxic glucose from the blood makes it good.

After a night's sleep, the hours that you've fasted have depleted the glucose stores in your liver. Your first meal replenishes some of these stores used up overnight. Once the stores are replete, any glucose that isn't burned in activity is converted and stored as fat.

Since OJ causes a rapid rise in insulin (the "insulin spike"), it also causes a rapid decrease in blood sugar levels. When this sugar is cleared quickly, you feel the "crash"—a swift decrease in energy level and increase in hunger. You feel tired, sluggish, and jittery, and begin to crave sweets. By this time, you have driven to work and started your day. Now you're hungry but didn't bring a snack.

However, your coworker and the vending machine down the hall both have a fine selection of sugary snacks. So you eat some of this sweet delight. Now your insulin spikes again, and the cycle of craving and crashing is perpetuated. You get to lunch with another valley in your blood sugar and you eat more than you should because you're even hungrier. When you're hungry and stressed from work, you subconsciously opt for calorie-rich comfort foods like pizza, pastas, burgers, and fries. More spikes occur throughout the day.

Over the years, this excess blood sugar and insulin can lead to a decrease in your body's sensitivity to insulin. It's like becoming tolerant of a drug. You need more sugar and insulin to get an effect. In fact, sugar really is a drug to which the body responds to much as it would to cocaine through the release of the neurotransmitter dopamine. The problem is, almost all of us are already addicted to sugar.

The body adapts to its environment. When something is thrown at it too much, it decreases its sensitivity. Your hands build up callouses when you work hard. Your muscles grow to avoid injury when you lift weights. Or worse, drug addicts need more and more pain medicine when they abuse a drug because they build up a tolerance. The intolerance to insulin, or insulin resistance, is a major factor in type 2 diabetes. This preventable form of diabetes is on the rise in our country and a major contributor to death and disability in America.

When you go to the grocery store and see juice products, they don't seem so healthy anymore, do they? We struggle with our diets because marketers and manufacturers take advantage of healthy connotations by overusing words like "juice." Juice is the Florida sun squeezed into a glass from healthy fruits, right? We struggle with food choices and we fail at our diets when it isn't necessarily our fault. We are misled down a path of "natural" and "wholesome" foods that ruin our goals to be lean and healthy.

If a manufacturer put "sugar" as a major ingredient on a product, many parents would shy away from that product. But many think, "Juice is better for my child. I know that OJ is healthy because it comes from fruit." Don't be distracted by such gibberish any longer! Just look at how Post Foods changed the name of one of its cereals from Sugar Crisp to Golden Crisp. Sugar obviously has unhealthy connotations, and the change in name helped boost sales. The focus of Post's advertising shifted from targeting just children to including parents by downplaying the sweet taste and associated sugar content.

WHEAT ADDICTION

Many of us are addicted to wheat, which is processed into breads, pastas, cakes, cookies, and breakfast cereals, and is even used as a thickening agent in other products like packaged soups. More than 700 million tons of wheat are produced globally each year.

Over the past century, wheat has been bred to provide favorable characteristics to not only wheat farmers but also food processors. Breeding more palatable wheat leading to greater consumption is obviously ideal for manufacturers. How about breeding wheat that contains more of an addictive substance so you eat and buy more? And I'm not talking about more sugar.

Wheat contains protein in the form of wheat gluten, which has a protein fraction called *gliadin*. Gliadin has some disturbing effects. In a 1979 study, scientists found that the gliadin fraction of gluten exhibited remarkably high "opioid-like" activity. This suggests that wheat gluten proteins may be addictive on their own despite our addiction to sugars. Furthermore, we know that the anti-opioid addiction medication, naltrexone, is prescribed to help with weight loss, possibly by inhibiting the appetite-stimulating effects of gluten. The author of *Wheat Belly*, Dr. William Davis, has suggested that cultivation and breeding of wheat has led to wheat containing more of these addictive proteins—to the advantage of food manufacturers. By using more addictive wheat in their products, manufacturers make greater profits because people eat more.

What does this mean for you? Processed foods that contain wheat flour are potentially addictive and can lead to unhealthy food choices that are hard to overcome. A recent popular push has been made to eliminate gluten from the diet because of potential adverse health effects. Some researchers have suggested that wheat proteins can cause leaky gut syndrome, which allows more allergens and pathogens to get into the body and causes a host of other problems such as autoimmune diseases and inflammation. The jury is still out on wheat, but the evidence points toward limiting it in your diet. Don't be fooled by the healthiness claims attributed to whole wheat and whole grains.

I can tell you firsthand that wheat and sugars *are* addictive. As a bodybuilder, I prepared for contests with extreme dieting to become as lean as possible. I would go on an extremely low-carbohydrate diet with sufficient protein and healthy fats to maintain muscle. The first 2 weeks of eliminating carbohydrates like wheat is mentally challenging. There are constant cravings and even symptoms of withdrawal such as extreme appetite, jitteriness, fatigue, and loss of concentration or focus. Once I made it through that brief period, my energy level stabilized, my focus improved, and I had less appetite than before starting. It is remarkable how well I would feel on a very low-carbohydrate diet. The drive of contest preparation makes the addiction easier to overcome, but finding that drive in everyday life is a challenge for all of us.

I will give you one more benefit of breaking the addiction to wheat. After you have been away from wheat for so long, the slightest bit becomes a delicacy. After contest prep, I would always taste the sweetness of foods a hundredfold. For example, a piece of white bread would have the flavor and pleasure of eating cake. In fact, a piece of real cake was almost intolerably sweet. Check with your doctor first, but I think we should all try a brief very low-carb diet to understand this phenomenon. It's an eye-opening experience.

What I realize looking back at this science and my own experience in cleansing myself of wheat addiction is that I needed to focus on the essential nutrients that won't fool the body and mind into becoming fat. We can live without bread and wheat-derived foods. We can achieve optimal physical and mental performance without sugar and carbohydrate-rich meals. We can eat healthy essential fats and have less worry about heart disease and obesity. We can take control of our food and activity to overcome our "bad genes." In fact, *The Leucine Factor Diet* will help you to feel your best every day while getting stronger and healthier.

CHAPTER 2

WHY LEUCINE?

The Leucine Factor Diet is all about the importance of leucine in our diets. Research and practical application have shown me that focusing on the leucine content of meals will optimize metabolic health and maintain muscle even through the toughest of fat-cutting diets. This diet will help you build muscle, get lean, and maintain metabolic currency.

Studies have shown that leucine activates mTOR, a signaling protein in cells that turns on muscle protein synthesis. They have also suggested that consuming between 0.04 and 0.05 grams of leucine per kilogram of body weight (or 0.02 grams per pound) per meal optimizes this effect of leucine on muscle growth, and that a minimum of 2 grams of leucine is needed to even partially activate muscle. This data seems to explain why the typical American diet of eating skewed protein where dinner is the central protein source does not optimize muscle protein synthesis throughout the day. Most Americans eat 10 grams of protein for breakfast, approximately

15 grams of protein for lunch, and 65 grams of protein for dinner. Even 10 grams of the highest quality protein doesn't come close to supplying 2 grams of leucine. The average 15 grams for lunch also fails to reach this threshold.

Leucine is one of the branched-chain amino acids (BCAAs), which are special because of their prevalence in muscle proteins. At one time gym goers and exercise scientists thought that we should consume more BCAAs just to improve our muscle structure and glycogen stores. Now it is becoming clearer through scientific discovery that the BCAA leucine allows muscles to use all of the essential amino acids more effectively.

In addition to acting as a signaling molecule to turn on mTOR, leucine is a critical component of what allows DNA to be read and duplicated. It is a component of proteins that help open up the DNA code called "leucine zippers." It appears that leucine is truly a special amino acid from the perspective of tissue remodeling, intracellular signaling, and activation of your genes.

Leucine has a noteworthy property that makes it ideal as a sensor of nutrient availability. It is one of the only amino acids (lysine being the other) that the body does not convert to glucose. The body can make glucose from proteins in a process called gluconeogenesis. Leucine is a non-gluconeogenic amino acid because it can't directly enter this process to become glucose.

During fasting or significant calorie restriction, the body tends to shift more protein into gluconeogenesis. Thus, amino acids consumed during this time may be more easily converted to glucose. Since leucine can't be converted to glucose, it retains its concentration in the blood proportionate with the food eaten. Thus, if you eat high-quality, leucine-rich protein, your body will have an accurate measure of how many nutrients you're bringing on board.

However, you can imagine that if you turn on mTOR without having the other essential amino acids available, you'll have a protein-making machine turned on but no other supplies to build the product. Even though leucine is a structural component of proteins, it isn't the only component. Thus, leucine doesn't work well on its own. Just taking leucine supplements won't cut it. Most proteins that are rich in leucine contain all of the essential amino acids, and a high leucine content is often a sign that the protein is high quality.

Researchers tested the hypothesis that the leucine content of a protein affects its ability to induce muscle protein synthesis. They compared wheat, soy, egg, and whey (soy has a higher leucine concentration than wheat, and egg higher than soy, and whey higher than egg). What they found was that relatively leucine-rich egg and whey showed significantly better performance than wheat or soy proteins, which naturally contain less leucine. When they added leucine to wheat, this difference decreased, supporting the importance of the leucine content of a meal in boosting muscle protein synthesis.

THE ANTI-SUGAR (ANTI-KRYPTONITE)

Because leucine is a non-gluconeogenic amino acid, the body can't directly convert it to glucose. That makes leucine essentially the anti-sugar agent. Leucine also has the ability to increase insulin release to push toxic sugars out of the blood.

The body's ability to handle sugar is often determined by obtaining a fasting blood glucose level. Elevated blood glucose is thought to represent insulin resistance and diabetes. However, rapid post-meal hyperglycemic spikes are thought to be of even greater consequence than fasting glucose levels in the development of cardiovascular disease.

The sugar consumed in a meal is not the only way to increase insulin release. Dietary protein and its digestion to amino acids like leucine have a very strong insulin-promoting effect to help clear toxic sugar. Consuming high-quality proteins rich in leucine with desired carbohydrates helps clear sugar from the blood. The less time that sugar stays in the blood, the less chance for tissue damage and inflammation.

Eat less sugar and more healthy proteins!

Animal and human studies show significant increases in insulin release with supplementing leucine to a protein and carbohydrate meal. Animal studies also show that leucine has the ability to increase the function and production of pancreatic cells that make insulin. This helps us to avoid the "burnout" of the pancreas, which can occur with metabolic syndrome and type 2 diabetes.

Another animal study examined the effects of adding leucine to the drinking water of mice fed a high-fat diet. After 14 weeks, the sensitivity of the mice to insulin improved by 50%. The researchers also noted nearly a 30% decrease in total cholesterol and more than 50% decrease in bad LDL cholesterol. In other words, in these mice the addition of leucine cured metabolic syndrome caused by an unhealthy diet.

PREVENTING MUSCLE BREAKDOWN

When it comes to staying strong like Superman or Superwoman, you must consider ways not only to build muscle but also to prevent its breakdown. This is particularly true when you cut back on calories and run the risk of breaking down muscle for fuel. Muscle is always in flux between breakdown and growth, much like many other tissues in the body.

The farming and the sports nutrition industries are always looking for the next metabolic jewel that can boost lean muscle mass for meat production or sports performance. Logically, breakdown products, or metabolites, of the powerful amino acid leucine have garnered the attention of scientists.

Beta-hydroxy-beta-methylbutyrate, or HMB, is the most popular of the leucine metabolites. In 1996, research by Professor Steven Nissen at my alma mater, Iowa State University, introduced HMB as a nutritional supplement. He showed that supplementation of up to 3 grams of HMB per day could partly prevent exercise-induced muscle damage, improve the amount of weight lifted, and build more muscle in healthy, young men lifting weights for the first time.

In 2013, the International Society of Sports Nutrition concluded that HMB supplementation can improve recovery from exercise, reducing muscle damage and enhancing muscle growth, strength, and power. It appears that HMB does this through prevention of muscle protein breakdown, more so than turning on muscle protein synthesis. In this way, the combination of leucine and HMB acts to build muscle and prevent its breakdown from stress (for example, from dieting, intense exercise, or immobility).

I have always recommended HMB and BCAAs to my clients trying to get leaner for bathing suit season, the contest stage, or weight-restricted sports. When you restrict calories to burn as much fat as possible or even to make weight, you are going to lose some muscle. It's the bodybuilder sparing the most muscle while burning the most fat who has the best chance to show up in the best condition with the most size. Studies have shown that HMB supplementation when training in a calorie-restricted state supports getting lean.

mTOR AND AGING

mTOR inhibition has been considered a way to prevent aging. In reality, as we age we lose muscle, have problems with balance and stability, and lose bone density partly because we lose sensitivity to leucine's ability to activate mTOR. Does it make sense to inhibit mTOR just because rats with low mTOR activity live longer?

mTOR and Muscle Mass

Muscle is metabolic currency and is thus metabolically expensive. When it comes to conservation of energy, muscle does the opposite. Muscle moves the body, constantly supports the skeleton, maintains body heat, and burns glucose. Nature needs a switch to know whether resources are plentiful enough to maintain this metabolically active tissue. The switch that turns on muscle protein synthesis (or maintenance of muscle mass) is mTOR.

With age, the body loses responsiveness to that signal to grow and develop. Elderly people need more leucine in their diets to turn on mTOR. Is the body saying it is time to slow down and wither away? I don't think so. Again, muscle is expensive to maintain and our aging body may just want to live off of retirement funds.

Many in the anti-aging medical community believe that mTOR causes us to age more quickly. I beg to differ. Animal studies suggest that inhibiting mTOR lets animals live longer. This often involves significantly restricting calories and limiting the stress on the animals. We don't live in a world without stressors and extreme low calorie diets just aren't sustainable. Our muscles need to respond, remodel, and grow to remain strong and active. mTOR activation helps us stay strong and keeps our skin, immune system, and other tissues healthy.

I argue the opposite. We should boost the leucine content of meals to avoid the complications of aging. Studies show that, in the elderly, supplementation with leucine and leucine-rich proteins like whey protein improve strength, mobility, and activities of daily living.

Furthermore, boosting sensitivity to leucine through vitamin D supplementation appears to reduce the risk of falls and improve metabolic health. Add HMB for the prevention of muscle loss with aging and we have a formula for strength and vitality into our golden years.

POWER OF THE SUN

Just as Superman received his power from the sun, so do all of us. Like our ancestors, we rely on the sun to fuel vegetation, and feed on nuts and vegetation as well as animals that ate the vegetation. The sun allows plants to produce oxygen for us to breath. Humans, animals, and plants could not be healthy without the energizing sun.

Our bodies respond to the sun, creating hormones like melatonin, which tells us when to sleep, and vitamin D, which builds our bones and muscles. Exposure to the sun promotes the formation of vitamin D in our skin. Vitamin D acts as a hormone that turns on genes controlling metabolism and growth. It is critical in turning on our muscles' sensitivity to the effects of insulin and leucine. In other words, we need the sun to make leucine work.

Over 40% of Americans and even more than this in my practice in Pittsburgh, where we get a little less sun than most, are vitamin D deficient. Some researchers have proposed a connection between vitamin D deficiency and the rising rates of diabetes and metabolic syndrome.

A lack of sun-derived vitamin D disrupts our metabolic health. Also, a lack of sun reduces feelings of motivation and positive mental attitude. Have you ever had the blues in the fall or winter? Feel great on that first sunny spring day? Changes in the seasons that result in less sun exposure can lead to depression and a condition called seasonal affective disorder, or SAD. The lack of motivation that ensues can derail any goals to get in shape. Further, vitamin D deficiency has been correlated to depression symptoms.

Other products of the sun are the nutrients provided by vegetation itself. Vegetables and fruits are rich in compounds called flavonoids and polyphenols that give them color and flavor. These compounds are biologically active with effects that we are just beginning to understand. They act as antioxidants to prevent free radical damage to our cells, which could otherwise lead to disease and cancer. They have biological actions that improve metabolism and increase insulin sensitivity in concert with leucine. The green leafy vegetables are particularly good at absorbing the power of the sun to create essential nutrients.

> Get out into the sun to improve your insulin and leucine sensitivity, metabolism, muscle function, bone density, and attitude!

DAIRY, WHEY TO GO!

"Drink your milk," my mom is always saying. However, milk consumption in the United States isn't what it used to be. Only 30% of adults get the recommended three servings of dairy per day. Furthermore, most Americans consume only 70% of the recommended amount of calcium per day, and many are vitamin D deficient.

Let's face it: America has a metabolic problem related to food choices and lack of exercise. Some of the fear of dairy consumption has arisen from the fat-free vogue, and dairy has been demonized by fad diet programs. I suggest that inactivity, overconsumption of sugar, and possibly a lack of dairy intake have led to an increase in the rate of metabolic syndrome among adults.

Amazingly, milk with its proteins and mineral content (calcium) has incredible effects on metabolism. Statistically, those who consume more than 35 servings of dairy per week have lessened their risk of developing metabolic syndrome by over 70%. Fortunately, exercise and dietary interventions can cure most cases of metabolic syndrome.

Randomized clinical trials of dairy consumption have demonstrated that increasing dairy intake to at least three servings from a single serving (or less) of dairy per day reduces waist circumference, blood pressure, and inflammation in overweight people. Dairy intake also improves insulin sensitivity. We don't yet know what part of dairy—calcium, protein, or vitamin D—improves health. More studies are in progress.

CALCIUM

Dairy products are a rich source of dietary calcium. For example, 1 cup of 1% milk contains about 300 milligrams of calcium. This is nearly one-third of the daily calcium requirement for most adults (approximately 1000 milligrams per day). Soybeans, kale, tree nuts, broccoli, arugula, sunflower seeds, white beans, bone-in sardines, salmon, and sesame seeds are all calcium-rich.

According to one theory, increased dietary calcium decreases the production of fat and directly stimulates fat breakdown. A review of research studies on calcium supplementation suggests that improved calcium intake (more than 800 milligrams per day) can improve body composition.

Calcium's most important role is in building strong bones, but it also plays a critical part in the action of our metabolic currency. The calcium stored in muscle is vital for muscle contraction and metabolism. Increasing the consumption of calcium-rich foods like low-fat dairy can improve metabolism and reduce body fat.

DAIRY PROTEINS

The main components of milk protein are whey and casein. Cow's milk is 80% casein and 20% whey. Whey protein is an incredibly rich source of leucine. Nature feeds us more whey (and thus more leucine) during the time we are growing the most, while breastfeeding. Human breast milk contains 60% whey protein and 40% casein. It would seem we are made to grow and develop in response to leucine-rich whey protein.

Milk proteins have incredible effects on health. For instance, digestion of milk proteins produces peptides that can reduce blood pressure and blood sugar. Studies of patients supplemented with milk proteins have shown significant reductions in both blood pressure and blood sugar nearly as effectively as some medications.

As very rich sources of leucine, milk proteins appear to provide much of the anti-kryptonite benefits of leucine discussed earlier. Milk proteins and specifically whey protein supplementation have been shown to improve insulin sensitivity and to lower post-meal blood sugar levels. Leucine clearly improves the development and maintenance of muscle mass. With more muscle comes more metabolic currency to overcome metabolic syndrome.

Anti-Kryptonite Benefits of Leucine

- Increases insulin release
- Pushes toxic sugars out of the blood
- Lowers post-meal blood sugar levels
- Improves development and maintenance of muscle mass

Whey protein enhances insulin action, and thus, the clearing of glucose from the blood. Science shows that adding 50 grams of whey protein to a carbohydrate meal effectively limits the rise in blood glucose levels through better insulin secretion and sensitivity. This effect would clearly be beneficial to people at risk for developing diabetes.

Along with glucose intolerance or insulin resistance, obesity is a major health concern. Obesity not only increases the risk for diabetes and heart disease, but is a major contributor to joint pain and disability as we age. One of the potential health benefits of whey protein is that it may suppress appetite more effectively than other forms of protein. The evidence for this effect is not quite as strong for obese individuals as it is for leaner people. Studies show that whey protein reduces hunger and increases metabolic rate better than other proteins like soy.

Another remarkably common condition in the aging population is high blood pressure, which can lead to cardiovascular disease and stroke. There are many different types of medications used to lower blood pressure when dietary modifications and exercise fail. These medications can be in the form of diuretics, beta-blockers, calcium channel blockers, or ACE inhibitors. When consumed daily, whey protein has been shown to decrease blood pressure almost as effectively as some of these medications. It appears to do this through the action of certain peptides (lactalbumin and lactoglobulin or lactokinins), which may act as inhibitors of ACE (angiotensin-converting enzyme), which produces a hormone that constricts blood vessels and elevates blood pressure.

This effect of whey protein on ACE is also of great interest to muscle builders in an indirect way, unrelated to its effect on blood pressure. The angiotensin II produced by ACE can lead to scarring of muscle after injury. We know that medication blocking angiotensin II improves muscle healing by increasing mTOR much as leucine does. The ACE inhibition and leucine activation that occur with whey proteins supports using whey protein for muscle growth.

Elevated triglycerides and cholesterol in the bloodstream increase the risk for heart disease and stroke. Adding 45 grams of whey protein to a typical meal decreases the elevation of triglycerides that occurs after that meal. Whey protein also limits systemic inflammation, which is caused by abdominal fat (belly fat) and has been linked to heart disease and cancer.

There is one other potential health benefit of whey protein that deserves mention. Whey protein provides some benefit by raising the levels of the antioxidant glutathione in the body. Glutathione protects cells from the actions of free radicals, which could potentially cause damage leading to inflammation and cancerous cell growth. Use whey protein to stay strong and healthy.

Mother's Milk

Mother's milk, or breast milk, helps us understand the importance of leucine in our diets. The milk contains 60% whey protein and 40% casein, compared with just 20% whey protein and 80% casein in cow's milk. This means that nature finds it more important to provide babies with leucine-rich whey protein than casein, which has a lower leucine content, for their growth and development.

ALL THE WAY WITH WHEY

Whey protein is so powerful in its ability to promote lean body mass, recovery from exercise, appetite control, and blood sugar control that it is an essential component of the Leucine Factor Diet. Not only do athletes benefit from whey protein's unique properties, but dieters, post-surgical patients, people with metabolic syndrome and diabetes, and otherwise malnourished individuals can benefit profoundly.

Whey protein is a rich source of highly bioavailable essential amino acids derived from the cheese-making process. Casein is a dense protein that is slowly absorbed. Whey protein is more rapidly absorbed, raising blood amino acid levels quickly after consumption.

Whey protein isolate has nearly 12% leucine compared with casein, which contains about 9%. It is this rich leucine content and proven health benefits that make whey protein an essential component of the Leucine Factor Diet.

Additionally, whey has a number of properties that are favorable. It improves immune system function and helps control blood pressure, appetite, and blood glucose. Additionally, whey protein is more effective gram for gram than soy and casein at enhancing muscle recovery from exercise in various studies.

WHEY VERSUS SOY

Scientists have recognized the differences among protein types and have done many studies on the effects of these proteins on body composition and recovery from resistance exercise like weight training. They have been particularly interested in comparing whey protein and soy protein.

The comparison has sparked interest because whey is from an animal source and soy is a plant. Many people believe the difference between these two proteins is related to the isoflavones found in soy, but research suggests otherwise.

Isoflavones = estrogen-like compounds with antioxidant properties found in legumes, also called "phyto" estrogens or "plant-derived" estrogens. Their health benefits are a subject of much debate in scientific literature. It is unclear how much effect soy isoflavones have on hormone physiology in men and women because of their estrogen-like activity.

A significant difference has been noted between whey and soy in their effects on muscle protein synthesis. One study showed that, at rest and after resistance exercise, consumption of whey protein produced an approximately 30% greater increase in muscle protein synthesis than soy protein. This correlates with the fact that whey protein contains nearly 30% more leucine than soy. Researchers suggest that this is a direct correlation. Your muscle's response to a protein is directly proportional to the leucine content of that protein.

Various types of whey protein are available, and each has pros and cons.

WHEY PROTEIN CONCENTRATE VERSUS ISOLATE

Whey protein concentrate, or WPC, is the rawest form of whey arising after removal from the milk-curdling process. The form of WPC usually sold contains 80% pure whey protein concentrate. The other 20% consists of lactose, fat, cholesterol, and minerals. Whey protein isolate, or WPI, is the purest form of whey protein; at 90% to 95% purity, it contains very little fat, lactose, or cholesterol. Because of its greater purity, WPI is more expensive than WPC. Cheaper protein supplements contain relatively inexpensive WPC, casein, and milk protein concentrates. The disadvantage of WPC is that you get less usable amino acids per gram of protein, and the lactose can cause intestinal discomfort in sensitive individuals. All WPCs are not created equal as well. Some may have a purity of 80% and others less, so consider the WPIs that must reach a 90% purity benchmark.

The best way to understand the quality of your protein supplement is to read the label. Greater amounts of sugar (lactose), cholesterol, and fat in the supplement may indicate that it is made from **WPC** rather than **WPI**, especially if the only ingredient is whey protein.

Whey protein contains microfractions of proteins including molecules like immunoglobulins (immune system–supporting proteins), alpha-lactalbumin and albumin, beta-lactoglobulin, glycomacropeptide, and lactoferrin. Whey protein concentrates are commonly extracted in a heat process that destroys these proteins. The high temperatures can also oxidize the cholesterol in WPC, making the cholesterol less healthy. Therefore, you may want to consider one of the following types of whey protein isolates:

Ion-exchanged whey protein isolates. Ion exchange is a purification process that concentrates the protein content while removing fat, lactose, and cholesterol. Ion-exchanged whey isolates are the purest of the whey proteins. However, the downside of this process is that it removes all the valuable and health-promoting microfraction peptides like immunoglobulins. Also, the process often leaves a high amount of beta-lactoglobulin, a common allergen in milk and may cause allergy issues in sensitive individuals.

Microfiltered whey protein isolates. Microfiltration produces very high-quality whey protein without destroying the microfractions that provide unique benefits to whey protein, such as support for the immune system and muscle-building potential. This type of whey protein is very low in fat, lactose, and cholesterol. Another upside to this form of whey protein is that it mixes easily in foods, shakes, and water with minimal clumping.

Hydrolyzed whey proteins. Hydrolysis is basically digestion of proteins into their individual amino acids. Whey protein can be treated enzymatically to create a "pre-digested" form of protein. This produces a more easily absorbed form of whey protein. Rapid absorption may be advantageous post-workout to get a quick rise in blood amino acid levels and stimulate recovery.

Research also shows that hydrolyzed whey promotes higher elevations of insulin than milk does. This augmentation of the insulin response by hydrolyzed whey is beneficial in controlling blood glucose and aiding in recovery from exercise. Small peptides of BCAAs from the digestion of whey may control insulin sensitivity and even blood pressure.

Is this an ideal protein for management of metabolic syndrome? Only further studies can answer that question.

PROTEIN AND HEALTH

Although the recommended daily allowance (RDA) is for only 0.8 grams per kilogram of body weight of protein per day, organizations like the American College of Sports Medicine and the International Society for Sports Nutrition have made it fairly clear in consensus statements that athletes need closer to 2 grams per kilogram of body weight per day. That is approximately 1 gram per pound of body weight per day.

MUSCLE PROTEIN SYNTHESIS

A 2014 study in the *Journal of Nutrition* also showed that most Americans tend to consume the majority of their protein in the evening meal. Most people eat approximately 10 grams at breakfast (for example, yogurt); approximately 15 grams at lunch (for example, chicken in a salad or lunch meat); and approximately 65 grams at dinner (for example, steak, fish, or chicken). Researchers decided to see what would happen to muscle protein synthesis if dietary protein were more evenly distributed across meals (30 grams x 3 meals). What they found was that evenly distributed protein led to more muscle protein synthesis. The threshold for muscle growth wasn't being reached with breakfast and lunch in diets where protein consumption was skewed toward dinner.

However, 30 grams of one type of protein may not have the same effect on muscle protein synthesis as another type of protein. Some researchers have shown that proteins like whey isolates have greater muscle growth responses than equal amounts of soy protein or wheat protein. It turns out that all proteins aren't created equal despite the fact that the RDA doesn't make this distinction.

The essential amino acids are the ones our bodies can't make. These amino acids must be consumed in order to form the proteins that allow us to survive. *Complete proteins* supply the body with all of the essential amino acids: leucine, phenylalanine, valine, threonine, tryptophan, methionine, isoleucine, lysine, and histidine. If a protein source is significantly deficient in just one of the essential amino acids, it is not considered complete. *Incomplete proteins* like lentils and wheat gluten lack certain essential amino acids; combinations of various incomplete proteins are required to form a complete protein.

BIOAVAILABILITY

Protein sources have a bioavailability rating that describes how well they break down into amino acids and how well those amino acids get absorbed into the bloodstream. If a protein source is not very bioavailable, then more of that protein will pass through the gastrointestinal tract and end up wasted in feces.

The goal in consuming extra protein is to get as many essential amino acids into the body in an efficient and cost-effective way. This can be done through highly digestible sources of protein like whey, egg, dairy, and soy. Supplemental sources of protein such as soy and whey are highly bioavailable.

The protein digestibility corrected amino acid score (PDCAAS) was established by the Food and Agriculture Organization of the United Nations in 1991 as a scoring method that assesses the amino acid composition of a protein relative to a reference amino acid pattern. That score is then corrected for differences in protein digestibility. The U.S. Dairy Export Council's Reference Manual for U.S. Whey and

Lactose Products rates whey protein isolate (derived from milk) as having the highest PDCAAS of all of the protein sources due to its high content of essential amino acids and BCAAs.

Casein, egg, and soy protein isolate are also classified as high-quality protein sources; all score 1.00 on the PDCAAS scale. Incomplete proteins like lentils and wheat gluten score 0.52 and 0.25, respectively. Notably, corn is very low in lysine and tryptophan, and thus is not a complete protein.

BENEFITS OF PROTEIN SUPPLEMENTATION

Scientific organizations like the American College of Sports Medicine and the International Society for Sports Nutrition feel that the RDA of 0.8 grams of protein per kilogram of body weight per day not only is insufficient but misrepresents the importance of protein in the American diet. Such a low amount of protein doesn't provide enough leucine.

Adequate protein intake is critical for maintaining lean muscle mass. Even non-athletes need lean muscle to maintain insulin sensitivity, metabolic rate, bone density, and strength for day-to-day activities. Ample protein protects the immune system and helps to heal the body from injury.

In 2004, researchers at Iowa State University, my alma mater, studied the effects of a placebo or a protein supplement given to Marine recruits after exercise. Although the supplement contained only 10 grams of protein, its effects were profound. After 54 days of basic training, the protein-consuming recruits had 33% fewer medical visits, including fewer viral and bacterial infections; 37% fewer orthopedic injuries; and 83% fewer visits due to heat exhaustion.

Additionally, the recruits using the supplement reported significantly less muscle soreness after training.

Animal studies have shown that whey protein has immune-enhancing properties. Human studies including the one at Iowa State University have proven that protein supplementation can help increase lean body mass, improve recovery after exercise, and support immune function during high-volume training periods (for example, twice-per-day training). This is especially true when proteins containing essential amino acids are consumed around training sessions.

SAFETY OF PROTEIN INTAKE

One of the biggest myths that the media and uninformed physicians, coaches, and parents spread is that "too much protein" (more than the recommended daily allowance of protein) leads to kidney and other medical problems. Even when I drink protein shakes at the hospital, other physicians ask me, "Aren't you worried about your kidneys?" I usually say, "Did you worry about going into renal failure with the fillet you ate at dinner last night?"

For some reason, the media has vilified sports supplements like protein shakes and creatine, and put them into the same category as anabolic steroids. They make them out to be an unfair advantage to athletes who consume them, and a health risk. The fact is that protein and creatine are beneficial nutrients found in red meat. By that logic, an athlete who eats a steak is cheating. In reality, protein and creatine supplements allow you to maintain a diet low in saturated fat and cholesterol by avoiding excessive intake of red meat.

The concern expressed is that high protein intake (by RDA standards) on a regular basis will result in overworking of the kidneys, which filter out the breakdown products of the protein consumed. Over time, the theory goes, this can lead to chronic kidney disease. The scientific evidence often cited comes from animal studies in which extraordinary levels of protein were fed or from human case reports of patients with preexisting kidney problems. It is a big stretch to apply these studies to a healthy person consuming extra protein.

When higher protein intake in healthy women without kidney disease was studied, no decline in kidney function was found. However, in women with mild kidney disease, higher consumption of protein, especially non-dairy protein, led to further decline in kidney function. Examined more closely, the decline in function might be related to fat or sodium content of processed meats and its effects on blood pressure rather than protein consumption.

Even vegetarians experience declines in kidney function as they age. Studies support the benefits of a relatively high protein diet in preventing diseases such as high blood pressure, diabetes, and metabolic syndrome, all of which predispose a person to kidney disease.

The International Society of Sports Nutrition acknowledges controversy over myths that high dietary protein intake can adversely affect bone metabolism. In reality, there are no studies that suggest a higher protein diet causes changes in bone density other than *improvement* when combined with an exercise program. The benefits of weight-bearing exercise on bone density are far greater than any theoretical bone loss from added protein intake. Increasing milk-based protein intake may be beneficial for improving calcium and vitamin D levels as well as promoting lean body mass, both of which support healthy bone density.

Despite individual metabolism and performance variables, I would like to make some steadfast recommendations about protein intake:

1. CONSUME MORE THAN ADEQUATE AMOUNTS OF PROTEIN.

Protein consumption is safe if you are healthy and have normal kidney function. The worst-case scenario is to lose hard-earned muscle because you are not consuming as much protein or leucine as you need. I recommend always consuming at least 1 gram of protein per pound of body weight per day.

2. CONSUME A VARIETY OF PROTEINS.

Variety is important in every aspect of life, including your diet and exercise. Consuming a variety of proteins such as fish, eggs, meat, and dairy will provide a range of micronutrients and fats that are essential for health, longevity, and performance.

3. TIME YOUR PROTEIN INTAKE.

Try to maintain a steady source of amino acids by eating meals about every 3 hours. (See the 5-MAD diet on page 52.) Spike your system with 3 to 6 grams of leucine (0.02 grams per pound of body weight per meal) by consuming high-quality protein such as a whey isolate before and after your workouts. This will maximize muscle protein synthesis and minimize breakdown.

4. CONSIDER A COMBO PROTEIN SUPPLEMENT WITH WHEY ISOLATES.

To boost your protein intake, first try microfiltered whey isolate. Not too expensive, it's relatively lactose-free, mixes easily, and is quite palatable as a shake or in oatmeal, Greek yogurt, or cooked foods. If affordable to you, a combo protein of microfiltered whey isolate and hydrolyzed whey is very palatable, mixes well, and has the advantage of rapid amino acid absorption with bi- and tripeptides that can be biologically active (improve insulin function and blood pressure). If the cost is prohibitive and you can tolerate lactose, fat, and cholesterol, whey protein concentrates still have the beneficial effects of BCAAs, microfractions, and easy digestibility of whey. If you choose soy protein, consider adding leucine or a BCAA blend to boost the effects on muscle protein synthesis.

5. ENDURANCE ATHLETES, YOU NEED PROTEIN TOO.

You are what you eat, and if you don't eat enough protein, you won't have enough muscle. Maintaining muscle mass is critical to the endurance athlete. Make sure to consume adequate amounts of muscle-sparing protein and energy-boosting carbohydrates and fats.

CHAPTER

3

THE THREE LEUCINE FACTOR LIFESTYLE GOALS

The Leucine Factor Diet was designed to help you achieve any or all of these goals: 1) maintain health, 2) build muscle, and 3) get lean.

MAINTAIN HEALTH: FIGHT AGING AT IDEAL BODY WEIGHT

If you feel that you are at your ideal body weight and you want to maintain that weight while living healthy for longevity, you are trying to maintain. You have reached the plateau of your desired weight and you are able to maintain it. Unfortunately, you need to realize that plateaus erode with time. Even though you may feel you are at an ideal body weight and in a healthy place, aging catches up with all of us. We need constant change if our bodies are to adapt to the environment. We need to introduce variety into our diets and exercise or we will fall back.

Nature and the human body both like efficiency; we don't like to waste energy or resources. The efficiency and balance of life is called *homeostasis*. This is a state of equilibrium so tightly controlled that small changes are easily accommodated and counterbalanced without shutting down the whole system.

In homeostasis, a rise in blood glucose triggers countermeasures such as the release of insulin by the pancreas to bring the glucose level back down. Blood pressure is tightly controlled by blood vessels, the kidneys, the heart, and compounds in the blood. Body temperature is so tightly controlled that when it rises significantly, we have no doubt that something has upset the applecart; illness has caused a fever.

Nature wants to be efficient in expending energy. It tries to conserve resources to avoid overtaxing the most important organ, the brain. Maintaining muscle requires a lot of energy as the tissue is very biologically active, whereas fat cells expend very little energy in storing energy. If you do not use your muscles, you will lose them, because the body would see them as useless consumers of valuable energy. It's like an efficiently run business. Why pay for a company car that sits in the parking lot all the time? You need to constantly prove to your body through challenging exercises that it needs to maintain its muscle and bone density.

Ill health results from imbalances in the body's homeostasis. Diseases and conditions like diabetes, dehydration, hypoglycemia, high blood pressure, obesity, gout, and any illness caused by a toxin disrupt homeostasis. That "toxin" can be sugar from the foods we eat disturbing pancreatic function; trans fat damaging blood vessel walls; lack of exercise weakening muscles and the heart; ultraviolet rays from the sun overpowering the skin's ability to repair DNA; lack of sleep overpowering the ability to stay awake; or even muscle breakdown products from training damaging the kidneys.

Under ideal circumstances, homeostatic control mechanisms should prevent imbalances from occurring. Unfortunately, in some people the mechanisms do not work efficiently enough or are overdepleted, or the quantity of toxins exceeds manageable levels. In these cases, medical intervention is necessary to restore balance, or permanent damage to organs may result.

How the Environment Affects Genes

Genes account for only a small portion of our health. The positive stimuli in our lives, such as restful sleep, as well as the negative ones, like mental stress, can affect the genes that are expressed and the viability of DNA.

Positive stimuli such as a healthy, antioxidant-rich diet and moderate- to high-intensity exercise can lead to the expression of genes to boost our metabolism, protect us from tissue damage, and improve our mental outlook. Negative physiological and mental stressors like smoking and interpersonal conflict can lead to the loss of healthy gene expression and further damage to DNA.

Our DNA is protected by little pieces of redundant DNA called telomeres. As we age, telomeres physically shorten and our DNA is at greater risk of damage. DNA damage leads to tissue breakdown, aging, and cancer. Telomeres last longer in people who do more than 3 hours of moderate exercise per week and avoid sugar and stress.

The body as a whole responds to stress much in the way that muscle does to exercise with transformation to accommodate future stress more efficiently. If you add a little stress (for example, from weightlifting), the homeostasis is slightly disturbed and the body brings balance to the system by producing new tissues or proteins so that it can accommodate that stress. Nonetheless, if you decide to do too much at once, the muscle will fail under the stress and tear. And if you decide to do too much too soon, the muscle won't have time to recover from the previous bout and will tear.

By recognizing the balance between stimulus (exercise, dietary changes) and recovery (sleep, stretching, cross-training, massage, supplements), we can maximize our efficiency in attaining our physical and mental goals. Balance needs to come into play in all aspects of our lives. Balance—between work and play, exercise and rest, sleeping and waking, impulse and aversion—leads to well-being.

The Leucine Factor Diet helps to bring balance to your muscles, mind, and metabolism by providing consistent leucine-containing food sources and occasional supplementation of leucine. As you have learned, all proteins are not created equal. Thus, even if you fulfill your protein consumption goals for the day, you may not be getting enough leucine at each meal to boost metabolism, control sugar, or maintain muscle. By introducing consistency in your leucine intake in a five-meals-a-day diet (5-MAD), the Leucine Factor Diet helps maintain metabolic homeostasis.

BUILD MUSCLE

For those who want to build muscle, like a physique athlete or bodybuilder, the Leucine Factor Diet gives you scientifically proven methods for building lean muscle and burning fat.

Muscle = Metabolic Currency. Muscle plays a bigger role in health than just looking good and providing strength. It is a complex metabolic machine that affects the entire body. The more muscle you have, the more metabolic machinery you have to burn fat and maintain the health of other organs like your brain.

That's right, building muscle helps build brain cells. Growing muscle cells release growth factors (small proteins that affect cells in the body much as hormones do) such as a protein called brain-derived neurotrophic factor, or BDNF. It crosses the blood–brain barrier and stimulates the formation of new brain cells. If you doubt the connection between muscle and brain health, keep in mind that research has shown over and over again that active kids do better in school.

The Leucine Factor Diet is all about building or at least maintaining muscle. Even those who just want to maintain their health have to fight the inevitable loss of muscle that occurs with aging. For those who want to burn fat, the goal is to maintain as much muscle as possible to keep their metabolism revved up.

Anabolism versus catabolism. Most tissue in your body, including muscle, is constantly remodeling. That is to say, your body is in a constant cycle of building up (anabolism) and breaking down (catabolism). Many of the cells in your body today are very different from the ones you had 10 years ago. Muscle responds to stress by adapting. If you lift heavier weights now than you used to, your muscle grows stronger. If you run for a longer time today than you did yesterday, your muscle generates more endurance capacity.

Muscle growth, or building up, requires an anabolic environment: adequate stimulus (exercise); anabolic hormones (for example, testosterone and insulin); and nutrients for growth (such as protein and leucine). All of these elements are required for maximum muscle growth.

One of the more neglected aspects of the cycle of muscle building up and breaking down is how anabolism and catabolism are always in balance. The goal of exercise, boosting hormones, and a high-protein diet is to maximize anabolism. There is also a need to limit catabolism. Stress and nutrient deficiencies result in increased catabolic hormones like cortisol, which break down muscle proteins. To grow muscle, you must increase anabolism while decreasing catabolism.

Through the Leucine Factor Diet plans, nutritional supplementation, stress management, and targeted exercise principles, you can minimize muscle breakdown or even build muscle while burning fat.

GET LEAN

If your goal is to lose excess fat, I suggest doing it while maintaining as much muscle as possible for strength and metabolic currency. You may be preparing for a physique competition or might need to make weight for a sport. Or you may simply want to lose weight because your doctor told you that you need to. Losing weight means that you'll burn fat and possibly lose some muscle. I want you to focus on burning fat more than losing body weight. With a proper diet and the right amount of exercise, you *will* burn fat.

Fat is the most abundant source of energy in our bodies. Most people have more than 10,000 calories of stored fat. There are two types of fat: white fat and brown fat. White fat, or white adipose tissue, is the fat that insulates your body and stores excess calories. Brown fat, or brown adipose tissue, is metabolically very active and helps maintain body temperature, especially when you are young. The objective is to enhance brown fat activity and burn white fat stores.

Your body constantly burns energy, even when you are sleeping or sitting. The energy expenditure of your body at rest is your basal metabolic rate (BMR; also called resting metabolic rate). Your BMR, which is measured as the number of calories per day your body burns at rest, can be estimated based on your height, weight, sex, and age. Every activity that you participate in adds calorie expenditure to your BMR. If your BMR is 1500 calories per day and you perform 500 calories of exercise during the day, your total daily expenditure (TDE) is 2000 calories.

Although BMR is routinely estimated with equations based on body surface area and lean muscle mass, it is important to realize that this is not an exact science. Individuals with the same lean body mass can have vastly different BMRs. One study showed a nearly 30% difference between two individuals of the same age, gender, height, and lean mass. This means that an estimate of the dietary calories you need daily requires careful follow-up of progress toward your goal. As you'll see throughout this book, I encourage constant grading of progress and adjustments as needed.

Your BMR is controlled by hormones released from the hypothalamus in your brain and from your autonomic nervous system. Thyroid hormone, epinephrine (adrenalin), and other hormones are important in maintaining BMR. A single exercise session can boost BMR throughout the day as well as burn fuel during the exercise. Building muscle helps boost BMR by accumulating more metabolic currency.

Creatine phosphate and glucose (stored in muscle as glycogen) are the most readily available energy sources for muscle. If glucose is prevalent, fat stays in its stores under the skin and in the belly. When you exercise, fast intermittently, or go on a low-carb diet, glucose becomes less available, and thus your body mobilizes fat from its stores to provide a source of energy. The body burns fat through a process called *beta-oxidation,* the most efficient way to produce energy. This is the process your body uses in an endurance challenge. If you have very low carbohydrate levels, your body will preferentially burn fat throughout the day by converting the stores to ketones (ketosis).

Your brain automatically monitors if there's enough food being consumed to keep your BMR up. If you are calorie restricted (on a low-calorie diet) your brain senses this and causes your BMR to decrease to avoid burning up valuable nutrients that keep the brain functioning. This "starvation response" kicks the body into storage mode.

A key principle of the Leucine Factor Diet is to avoid ever going into this fat storage mode. The diet is based on a number of scientific principles intended to maximize lean muscle mass while losing fat or beefing up. The objective, always, is to stay anabolic and maintain your muscle as metabolic currency. Although losing weight is largely a catabolic process, anabolic stimuli can help you to maintain muscle while losing fat.

4

TIMING IS EVERYTHING

Nutrient timing is a critical component of the Leucine Factor Diet plan. Your metabolism is regulated by a system of clocks in your brain and your body. Hormones and nutrient assimilation from food are controlled by the light-dark/waking-sleeping cycles called circadian rhythms. Disruption of the regularity of these rhythms results in metabolic dysfunction and chronic lifestyle diseases like obesity, diabetes, and heart disease. One of the best examples of this is the high rate of metabolic syndrome in people with shift-work sleep disorders.

The "brain clock" responds to the light and dark cycles that control the main regulators of hormone release in the hypothalamus and pituitary gland. For instance, darkness induces melatonin release and the initiation of sleep, followed by the release of growth hormone in the deepest stages of sleep. The "body clock" responds to nutrient intake and controls metabolism through hormones like insulin. If your nutrient timing is catawampus, your body clock will spiral out of control, leading to insulin resistance and metabolic dysfunction.

GET REGULAR SLEEP

Consistency is the key in keeping your internal clocks working like Swiss timepieces. It is the most important aspect of nutrient timing for muscle growth. You need to be consistent in the times that you go to sleep and wake up. With a regular sleep schedule, you can optimize recovery from training and release of anabolic hormones like growth hormone. And with a consistent meal schedule, your metabolism can stop guessing when nutrients will be available to build muscle. Consistency avoids overstorage and starvation responses that can lead to packing on fat for survival in the famine.

When your goal is to build or maintain lean muscle, you need to optimize muscle anabolism while limiting muscle catabolism. Intense training in the gym results in the breakdown of muscle proteins along with the stored nutrients like glycogen. Timing of nutrient intake can help limit excessive muscle breakdown and optimize the utilization of resources for muscle growth. Also, timing of nutrient intake can affect performance in the gym. With proper timing, you can boost workout intensity and recovery from set to set.

THE ANABOLIC WINDOW

There is a big debate in sports nutrition literature about how long the "anabolic window" after exercise remains open. This is the period in which muscle is more responsive to protein consumption for building more muscle protein.

It was originally thought that muscle was most responsive to protein within the first 1 to 2 hours after exercise. However, research suggests that muscle may be responsive to the stimulatory effects of protein and leucine for over 24 hours. The idea that you need to consume rapidly absorbed carbohydrates after training for the purpose of getting an insulin spike to boost anabolism has been debunked by scientific literature. In fact, the essential amino acids provide enough stimulus of muscle protein synthesis that sugars and insulin aren't needed. That being said, there is some logic I would like to interject into the timing of your meals.

It makes sense to me that you would want to consume rapidly absorbed protein around the time of your workout for a number of reasons. First, increased blood flow to working muscles, which are very receptive to absorbing nutrients, occurs after training. If you consume some protein before your training, amino acids will be available to enter the muscle when the blood flow to the trained muscle increases. Second, intense training can lead to an initial catabolic response in muscle. This is an initial breakdown of muscle before the buildup in recovery. Amino acids like leucine and HMB are great at limiting that muscle catabolism and boosting the synthesis process. Why not nip catabolism in the bud by having amino acids available immediately before as well as after your exercise.

Even though a couple of studies found it doesn't matter when you get your protein in relation to your exercise, those studies didn't say that having protein close to your workout was detrimental. On the other hand, a few studies have shown that consuming protein immediately before or after your workout is associated with a greater rise in muscle protein synthesis than having the same protein in the morning and evening. Since there are no disadvantages, and possible advantages, why not just consume protein before and/or immediately after your training?

My recommendation is that you consume high-quality protein like whey isolates within 30 minutes before and 30 minutes after your training. The protein that you use before and after should provide your minimum total leucine requirements per meal. For example, if you need 40 grams of whey to get your leucine needs, consume 20 grams before your workout and 20 grams after. If you aren't worried about burning fat and want to build muscle, feel free to add an equal amount of carbohydrates to each of the pre- and post-workout meals.

THE FIVE-MEALS-A-DAY PLAN (5-MAD)

Your body needs a consistent supply of nutrients to build and recover from intense exercise. The typical three meals per day of breakfast, lunch, and dinner just don't fit our physiology. Even if you have a substantial breakfast, you are probably very hungry by the time lunch comes around. Somewhere along the way you may have had a snack to quench those hunger pangs. Often, that snack is some overprocessed, sugar-laden, malnutritious food, just to tide you over.

In reality, that snack just made things worse for lunch. The highly processed and rapidly absorbed carbohydrates in a sugary snack produce an insulin surge, which causes a rapid decline in blood glucose and a surge in appetite. It's the same thing that happens when you drink juice (see OJ Conundrum, page 13). You go to lunch with a desire to eat as much if not more food than you would have without the additional appetite surge, and you end up with a post-lunch slump in energy. This is a vicious cycle that can be broken by rethinking your eating schedule.

I suggest that you adopt the five-meals-a-day plan (5-MAD) to stabilize blood glucose levels and supply your muscle with quality nutrients and leucine throughout the day. Studies on maximizing muscle protein synthesis with a balanced feeding schedule in critically ill patients suggest meals every 3 hours. The importance of low-glycemic carbohydrates, high-quality proteins, and essential fatty acids will be discussed later; but each meal should provide these while also supplying fiber and antioxidants, preferably from nuts and vegetables. More important, each meal should contain essential nutrients that you can't live without. Again, there are essential amino acids in protein, essential fatty acids in fats, and essential vitamins and minerals in nutrient-dense foods. There are no essential carbohydrates, other than fiber, so starches and sugars are not absolutely necessary in every meal.

In sports training or for those just trying to lose body fat, meal frequency and nutrient timing are critical. The typical three meals per day—breakfast, lunch, and dinner—just don't cut it when trying to maximize performance or metabolism. Depending on how long your day is, a three-meals-a-day plan leads to excessive periods without fuel to recover and maintain or build muscle.

During infancy, babies tend to eat throughout the day. Have you noticed how quickly babies double their body weight and size? They are growing rapidly by consuming leucine-rich human milk protein on a more frequent schedule than three meals a day. If you want to put on muscle, eat more like a baby, regularly, with a leucine-rich meal!

Some people think that increasing meal frequency without changes in total daily calorie intake can increase metabolic rate and fat burning, but this isn't supported by the scientific literature. However, if your leucine intake is adequate, increased meal frequency can help you spare muscle mass when you're on an energy-deficient, fat-burning program—that is, when you expend more calories than you take in. Smaller meals may also improve your muscle's effectiveness in burning fat because less insulin is released at any given meal. Insulin shuts down fat burning and switches on fat storage.

A snack between meals has actually been shown to burn more body fat and improve strength despite small increases in total calories consumed. Beyond the muscle-sparing effects of eating more than three meals a day, the increase in frequency of protein consumption may improve appetite control. When I say "eating more than three meals a day," I do not mean that you eat your usual three meals and add meals on top of that so that you eat more calories—although you might do that if your goal is to gain weight. But when you are trying to improve performance or burn fat, the goal is to maximize the effects of meal frequency in limiting muscle breakdown by eating foods that deliver needed leucine without excessive calories.

An increase in meal frequency also has a beneficial effect on blood markers of health such as cholesterol and even decreases blood pressure. Eating more than four meals a day, with the same total calories as someone eating three meals a day, can lead to lower total and bad LDL cholesterol levels. The effect is almost as strong as some medications for high cholesterol. Furthermore, with smaller meals comes lower levels of blood glucose, less "caramelizing" of tissues, and thus, less total body inflammation.

PERI-WORKOUT NUTRITION

Peri-workout nutrition means consuming nutrients before, during, or after your training. Supplementation with a shake containing protein, carbohydrate, and creatine increases lean body mass, strength, muscle size, and muscle creatine and glycogen levels. A study by Australian scientists demonstrated a profound benefit to supplementing these nutrients immediately before and after a workout rather than in the morning and evening (not immediately around the workout time).

Scientists have demonstrated that consuming supplements containing carbohydrate, fat, and protein (chocolate milk, for instance) within 30 minutes before exercise can improve vertical jump power and number of repetitions of high-intensity resistance training.

Caffeine is another aspect of peri-workout nutrition that deserves recognition. Consumed prior to exercise or competition, caffeine is very effective in improving performance in endurance exercise and high-intensity intermittent exercise like soccer or rugby. Caffeine can even boost concentration during exercise and recovery from training. It is effective at moderate doses of approximately 2 milligrams per pound of body weight (about as much as a 16-ounce bold coffee).

One fear about caffeine is that it may have a diuretic or water-wasting effect that can lead to dehydration and poor performance. However, this effect is not supported by the scientific literature, and caffeine use appears to be safe. Sensitivity to caffeine from coffee or other sources can wane over continued use (i.e., it takes more to keep you awake than before). It may be beneficial to give your body a break from caffeine on occasion in order to improve its performance-enhancing effects.

Consuming BCAAs and/or HMB before fasted cardio (page 137) can help spare muscle. Science supports that BCAA supplementation improves fat burning during glycogen-depleted cardio. This is cardio exercise when your muscles are empty of any sugar stores for energy. When your sugar stores are depleted, you run the risk of burning muscle protein for energy. Thus, I recommend consuming added leucine and BCAAs prior to fasted morning cardio to protect your muscle.

INTERMITTENT FASTING VERSUS CHRONIC CALORIE RESTRICTION

Modern humans are still genetically adapted to a preagricultural hunter-gatherer lifestyle. Our overall genetic makeup has changed very little in the past 10,000 years. Hunter-gatherer societies likely engaged in moderate physical activity for more than the currently recommended 30 minutes each day, to provide basic necessities for survival, such as food, water, shelter, and fuel for fire.

You might think that any gene that didn't support an active lifestyle would have died off through natural selection. By the same logic, a gene that supported physical activity even in times of famine would have survived, and its gene pool inherited by future generations. Thus, it is likely that many metabolic functions of modern humans evolved as adaptations to a physically active lifestyle that was, coupled with a diet high in protein and low in carbohydrate, interspersed with frequent periods of famine.

The concept of cycles of feast and famine in our ancestors engendered the "thrifty gene" hypothesis. According to this hypothesis, individuals with thrifty metabolic adaptations convert more of their calories into fat during periods of feasting. As a consequence, those with the thrifty genes are less likely to die off during food shortages because they have better fat stores. This theory certainly has its critics in that we really don't know for certain how our ancestors lived, but it helps us to understand some of our physiology, as we will discuss.

A reduction in energy intake to a level less than your body requires for basic functions and activity results in a series of physiological, biochemical, and behavioral responses, which are adaptations to the low-energy intake. Once the body burns off all of its stored glucose (glycogen), it starts to burn fat for energy. In times of prolonged energy restriction, muscle breaks down into amino acids that can be used for energy production. Furthermore, when your energy intake is low, you become less active and your metabolism slows down. Inactivity produces muscle atrophy, which then culminates in even less metabolic activity.

When you chronically restrict your diet, as in a weight-loss program, you turn on some of these adaptive responses. Your metabolism has a tendency to slow down, you stop building muscle or even lose muscle, and you are more inclined to store extra food as fat. You may become a yo-yo dieter. When you restrict food for a significant period of time, you lose muscle, which acts as metabolic currency. The more muscle you have, the more fat-burning potential. When dieters who have lost muscle go back to eating more than they need, they end up storing more fat because the fat becomes a sponge and the muscle is gone.

Many people now realize that chronically restricting calories is probably not the best way to burn fat. Although some animal studies suggest that lower energy intake leads to longer life, this has yet to be convincingly proved outside the laboratory or in humans. Chronic calorie restriction leads to hormonal changes, reduced muscle mass, lower bone density, increased risk of infection, susceptibility to physiological stress, and increases in appetite. Intermittent calorie restriction has been shown to be much more effective than chronic restriction in maintaining lean muscle mass in dieters. This is where the concept of intermittent fasting comes into play.

In preparing for contests, I always used intermittent fasting to burn fat while sparing my muscle mass. I did this through a high-protein, low-carbohydrate diet with healthy fats and fasted morning cardio exercise. By avoiding carbs in my last two meals and sleeping for 8 hours (essentially an overnight fast), my glycogen stores were at minimal levels by morning. By doing fat-burning cardio in this state, my body had to search for other sources of energy than stored glucose. The body's next preference is to burn fat, but muscle can be broken down to use as an energy source. However, with use of muscle-sparing supplements like BCAAs and HMB, I burned fat while maintaining my muscle.

Intermittent fasting (IF) comes in many forms. One IF technique involves an entire day of fasting, with only tea, coffee, and water allowed, but I don't encourage it as this is way too long to go without the muscle-activating effects of leucine. Another technique is to schedule significantly energy-restricted days twice weekly, when you eat a small amount of food containing less than 50 grams of carbohydrates. Yet another technique is to fast for the first half of the day and to work out during the fast. Another technique is to eat only during a 6- to 8-hour window during the day.

IF puts the body on notice that glucose won't always be available to burn for fuel. In diets where you eat throughout the day with the typical recommended daily allowance emphasizing carbs over protein and fats, the body is constantly using glucose for fuel. By fasting, you encourage fat-burning machinery to stay active and ready to mobilize fat from its stores. IF has been scientifically proven to be as effective, if not more effective, than chronically calorie-restricted diets in helping subjects lose weight and restore insulin sensitivity.

IF seems to restore normal physiology in overweight people. It also improves blood triglyceride and cholesterol levels, further reducing the risk of heart disease. Short episodes of fasting help train your body to deal with stress. Exercise and fasting affect physiology in similar ways. By forcing your body to use another source of energy (that is, fat), IF trains your body to burn fat more efficiently. The metabolic engines of your muscle respond to stress much as they respond to weight training. If you stress muscles by lifting heavy weights, those muscles tend to grow. However, if you overstress muscles with too much weight, you induce an overload that can do more harm than good. Thus, proponents of IF don't suggest that you fast forever, but that you do it in small bursts.

IF also seems to normalize other hormones. Growth hormone is a restorative hormone released in response to exercise and sleep. It plays a role in conserving muscle mass while also maintaining blood glucose levels and mobilizing fat to be burned. Fasting has been shown to temporarily raise growth hormone levels by as much as 1300% in women and 2000% in men.

In addition, IF normalizes hormones that lead to hunger, making it less difficult to deal with the lack of food. In particular, studies show that the "hunger hormone" ghrelin is reduced by IF.

One more benefit that is worth mentioning is the effect of fasting on the brain. The brains of animals stressed by a lack of food become more active to help those animals focus on finding food. Furthermore, the brain likes ketones that arise from the breakdown of fat for fuel. A study showed that alternate day fasting in which subjects consume only 600 calories in one meal on the fasting day increases brain-derived neurotrophic factor (BDNF) by up to 400%. BDNF is involved in the growth of new brain cells and learning. Studies also show that exercise is associated with similar increases in BDNF. This elevation in BDNF is also thought to be protective in cognitive diseases like Alzheimer's. In animal models, IF can delay the onset of memory disorders like Alzheimer's. Whether this effect occurs in humans is yet to be studied.

> Ketones are compounds derived from fats or amino acids in the body that can act as a fuel source for our brains and hearts. They become more available during times of fasting and very low-carbohydrate dieting.

If all of this convinces you to try intermittent fasting, you are in for a challenge. Most studies of IF have a pretty high attrition rate. This means that the diets were very difficult to follow and many test subjects just couldn't hack it for the full 12-week study.

I recommend starting with a 5:2 diet. This is 5 days of regular eating interspersed with 2 days of eating only a calorie-restricted afternoon meal. For instance, you eat basically what you want for 5 normal days at 2000 calories, and then eat only 600 calories for one afternoon meal for 2 non-consecutive days interspersed in the week. Consult with your physician before trying any new diet routine, especially one this radical.

I don't believe a full fast of no food, as many IFers suggest, is necessary to get the effects of fasting metabolism. Low-carbohydrate, high-protein meals timed around your exercise can have similar effects on your physiology. Try doing fasted morning cardio and train with weights in the afternoon after you have had a couple of meals and a pre-workout shake. Take BCAAs and HMB to help spare muscle, and keep your protein intake up to at least 1 gram per pound of body weight. Eat a well-balanced diet with vegetables, fish, meat, eggs, nuts, and dairy—or just go paleo if you want to live like your cave-dwelling ancestors!

5

ALL CALORIES ARE NOT CREATED EQUAL

True, a calorie is a calorie—but the different sources of calories can affect the body differently. As you can imagine, since this book is about the anti-kryptonite power of the essential nutrient leucine, all calories are absolutely not created equal. Leucine has powerful metabolic properties despite its available 4 calories per gram. Leucine is an amino acid found in proteins, which means that it can be a source of calories for the body. However, 1 gram of leucine has significantly more power as a nutrient than 1 gram of sugar even though they contain the same number of burnable calories.

THE ESSENTIAL MACRONUTRIENTS

Macronutrients are the fats, carbohydrates, and proteins that are our main sources of energy (calories) and tissue structure. These aren't to be confused with micronutrients such as vitamins and minerals, which are nutrients without calories consumed in small quantities. Of the three macronutrients, only two are essential in our diet: essential fats and essential amino acids.

ESSENTIAL FATS

Certain fats are called "essential fats" because we can't survive without them, but our bodies can't make them. The essential fats include *alpha-linolenic acid* (ALA; an omega-3 fatty acid) and *linoleic acid* (an omega-6 fatty acid). They not only act as energy sources, but they also provide structure to cell membranes and nerve linings, and are precursors of prostaglandins, which can rebuild tissues and even cause pain. Knowing this, does it make sense to live on a fat-free diet?

To suggest that we should live fat-free is an oversimplification of the fact that most Americans need to consume fewer calories, no matter their origin. Since fats are calorie rich at 9 calories per gram compared with 4 calories per gram for proteins and carbohydrates, dieters often limit them first. However, the focus should be on limiting sugar and other carbohydrates, and replacing saturated animal fats with healthier fats like omega-3 fish oil and monounsaturated fats from nuts.

In general, fats improve digestion. They delay the emptying of food from the stomach just as bulky fiber does. Fat-containing foods sit in the stomach longer and are better digested. The slowdown in digestion causes ingested sugars to reach the blood more slowly. This means that fats reduce the rapid rise in blood sugar that leads to insulin resistance in type 2 diabetes. Certain fats have greater ability to reduce appetite than others, such as fish oils.

In addition to having different digestive properties, fats also vary in their effects on the body. Fats aren't just sources of calories and insulation. They are essential for the health of nerves, skin, muscle, brain, heart, and more. Fats and cholesterol also make up the membranes of cells throughout the body, and different fats have various effects on the fluidity of those membranes. From the fats in the membranes, cells make inflammatory mediators like prostaglandins, which play critical roles in tissue repair and inflammation.

> The nonsteroidal anti-inflammatory drugs (NSAIDs) like ibuprofen and naproxen inhibit the production of prostaglandins. Prostaglandins cause fever, pain, and swelling. However, they also initiate healing and improve blood flow and control bleeding. These processes are essential to good health. Limit your use of NSAIDs and ask your physician for guidance.

Fats are incorporated into *triglycerides,* which are stored in fat cells and carried in the blood with cholesterol and lipoproteins. Triglycerides can be produced from dietary fat or fat produced by the liver from excess sugar. Excess triglycerides in your blood is considered a significant risk factor for heart disease.

Unsaturated fat comes in two forms: polyunsaturated fatty acids (PUFAs) and monounsaturated fatty acids (MUFAs). These fats are often considered the "healthy" fats in our diets as studies have shown their beneficial effects in comparison to diets high in saturated fats. The short-chain fatty acids that you can't live without are PUFAs, including omega-3s and omega-6s. These essential fatty acids are the foundation of long-chain polyunsaturated fatty acids, or LC-PUFAs, which are common in fish oil. LC-PUFAs have very important biological effects on heart, brain, and total body health. That being said, LC-PUFAs are not essential if short-chain PUFAs are available. But this gets tricky.

The short-chain PUFAs that we consume as omega-3s and omega-6s can be elongated to LC-PUFAs in the body, but our enzymes are very inefficient at performing this task. Fortunately, microalgae in the ocean are much more adept at doing this than humans. They suck up energy from the sun and convert it into fatty acids that fish consume.

The omega-3 LC-PUFAs are much easier to get from fish whose main diet is algae. Fish oil is the best source of eicosapentaenoic acid (EPA) and docosahexaenoic acid (DHA). EPA and DHA have physiological roles in the body that lead to better brain function, improved cardiovascular health, decreased inflammation, and improved insulin sensitivity. On the other hand, meats are rich in the omega-6 LC-PUFA called arachidonic acid. These fats, the omega-6s, are potentially more inflammatory but still provide an essential role and should not be neglected and vilified.

ESSENTIAL FATS FOR GOAL ATTAINMENT

Many studies indicate that the essential fats in fish oil have the potential to augment recovery from training in the gym, improve muscle building, and burn fat. Athletes have been known to take fish oil supplements to reduce body fat, increase lean muscle mass, and reduce muscle damage and inflammation. What does the science really say?

There are some theoretical as well as realized effects of increasing the consumption of fish oil from food or as a supplement. The main premise behind fish oil consumption is that the oil has an anti-inflammatory effect that can help limit soreness and get you mobile quicker. Multiple studies, in fact, do demonstrate that fish oil supplementation can reduce post-exercise inflammation and muscle soreness. Omega-6 fatty acids have a pro-inflammatory effect, so consuming more omega-3 fish oil tips the scales toward an anti-inflammatory environment in your body. When you are building your diet, consider using grass-fed meats and organic, free-range eggs that tend to have more omega-3 fats than your typical meats and poultry. Consider having a fish like salmon each day.

Red blood cells are more flexible and use oxygen more efficiently when omega-3s are integrated into their cell membranes More flexibility means that the red blood cells can squeeze through very small blood vessels in higher concentration and carry more oxygen to muscles. One study demonstrated that 6 grams of fish oil supplementation per day for 6 weeks resulted in enhanced oxygen delivery and maximal oxygen uptake during low oxygen high-altitude training.

Fish oil has also been shown to increase fat oxidation, reduce body weight, and prevent weight gain in laboratory animals. This basic science and further clinical data are quite convincing in that these essential fatty acids are beneficial to your health and will help you achieve your body composition goals.

OTHER FATTY ACIDS

Flax seed oil. This oil has a high proportion of omega-3 fatty acids in the form of short chains. However, your body can convert only a small percentage of short-chain fats into the more beneficial long-chain EPA and DHA found in fish oil. There is no need to supplement with flax oil; in fact, it would be a waste of money for that purpose. Use flax as a healthier oil for fat calories or flavor over vegetable oils if so desired.

Krill oil. In a few studies, krill oil was asserted to have beneficial effects similar to fish oil. It is derived from shrimp-like organisms found in large quantities in the ocean. A great source of omega-3 fatty acids, krill oil has anti-inflammatory effects and cardioprotective benefits similar to those of fish oil despite having approximately 60%

of the EPA and DHA found in fish oil. This suggests that the body may absorb krill oil better than fish oil.

CLA. Conjugated linoleic acid, or CLA, is another fatty acid that has great results in laboratory animals, with a few good human trials. The claim is that CLA supplementation's benefit is in helping to burn fat. Human studies have demonstrated that CLA supplementation improves endurance exercise performance and body composition (lower body fat percentage). However, there are conflicting human studies that have failed to demonstrate this effect.

Safflower oil. This oil made headlines when Doctor Oz touted its potential to promote weight loss. Safflower oil is rich in the essential omega-6 fatty acid, linoleic acid (it is approximately 78% linoleic acid). Studies show that this oil may be more effective than CLA in reducing belly fat and increasing lean mass. However, another study in which safflower oil replaced saturated fats in the diet showed increased rates of death from heart disease. Definitely food for thought, but I would not recommend adding safflower oil to your diet without further evidence. Use it in moderation if you like it for flavor.

Arachidonic acid. This pro-inflammatory omega-6 fatty acid is thought to be beneficial for muscle building by stimulating the production of muscle proteins, in much the same way that leucine does. Non-steroidal anti-inflammatory drugs, or NSAIDs, like ibuprofen and naproxen, which prevent formation of prostaglandins from arachidonic acid, can also stunt muscle growth and repair. Studies have shown significant improvement in sprinting speed with arachidonic acid supplementation. Also, data suggests that the prostaglandins made from arachidonic acid are able to increase muscle growth via receptors interacting through the same pathway as leucine, the mTOR pathway (refer to page 24).

PISSING IN THE OCEAN?

Clearly, there can be too little or too much of a good thing, and finding just the right balance is a challenge. Although all the fatty acids discussed here have the potential to improve your health and performance, supplementation will have little effect if your diet is out of whack.

A typical diet has an omega-6 to omega-3 ratio of more than 10 to 1. Some scientists theorize that humans may have evolved with a diet that had equal portions of those fatty acids. For health and longevity, the optimum ratio of omega-6 to omega-3 is thought to be 4 to 1 or lower. If your diet is out of whack, taking 2 grams of fish oil per day in a capsule or pill may not be enough to affect your ratio; it may be like pissing in the ocean, the omega-3 fats being overshadowed by the omega-6 and saturated fats. Taking more fish oil pills is definitely not the answer, but following the healthy Leucine Factor Diet is. I suggest that you begin with a clean diet: a combination of fish, lean grass-fed meats or dairy, and nuts. Then augment with desired fatty acids like fish oil.

NONESSENTIAL FATS

SATURATED FATS

This is the most energy-rich fat that solidifies at room temperature like lard. Saturated fatty acids are considered the bad fats. Clearly, lard and butter are not good for you. Multiple studies have correlated high saturated fat intake with higher rates of cardiovascular disease. Older studies provided evidence for replacing saturated fats with PUFAs to reduce risk of heart disease. However, recent studies suggest that saturated fat may not be as bad as once thought. This is science that is definitely in flux.

In your blood work, high total cholesterol, high LDL (bad cholesterol), and low HDL (good cholesterol) correlate to increased risk of heart disease, the number one killer in the country. There is very strong evidence that high saturated fat intake leads to higher total cholesterol, higher triglycerides, and higher LDL levels. Other studies have correlated high intake of saturated fats with cancer and bone disease.

Knowing that saturated fats contribute to cardiovascular disease risk, manufacturers have been replacing fats in foods with refined simple sugars. Unfortunately, removing fat from foods also removes some of the healthy fats. Increases in unhealthy sugars and decreases in health-promoting essential fatty acids constitute a double whammy. The main thing to learn from studies on saturated fats is to consume these fats only in moderation and to include healthy essential fatty acids, like fish oil and monounsaturated fats, in a well-balanced diet. That means avoiding processed meats and desserts or snacks and making fish, nuts, avocado, and olive oil part of your diet.

> The American Heart Association recommends limiting saturated fat intake to less than 10% of daily calories, and even less in high-risk individuals (for example, those with obesity, diabetes, family history of heart disease, and smokers).

Saturated fats, trans fat, and dietary cholesterol can raise blood cholesterol. Monounsaturated fats and polyunsaturated fats do not appear to raise the level of bad LDL cholesterol—and studies even suggest that they may help lower LDL cholesterol when consumed as part of a diet low in saturated fats and trans fat.

One other aspect of saturated fat consumption is the effect of carbohydrate on the way the body handles saturated fats. Multiple studies show that if you consume saturated fats on a low-carbohydrate diet, your LDL and blood triglycerides do not rise. It appears that carbohydrates cause more of the saturated fats to be stored rather than used for energy. In other words, sugars make you store saturated fat in your fat cells; they make you fatter. Saturated fats consumed in the form of meat, but without carbohydrate, have much less ability to make you fat. So the jury is still out on how bad saturated fats are for health. It may be the toxic sugars rather than the saturated fats creating the bad blood.

TRANS FAT

During food processing, unsaturated oils such as vegetable oils can be subjected to a process called hydrogenation to make them more solid at room temperature like saturated fats such as butter and lard. These partially hydrogenated oils are common in margarine and shortening. Once hydrogenated, the oils act like saturated fats, raising cholesterol levels in the blood. However, the chemical processing of the fats is even more damaging to health than saturated fats from animal sources. Trans fat causes inflammation that destroys blood vessel walls, leading to cardiovascular disease. Trans fat content is currently mandated on food labels, and consumption should be limited because of a correlation between trans fat and heart disease risk. Beware, trans fat is found in many chips, cookies, and other processed treats.

The American Heart Association recommends limiting trans fat intake to less than 1% of daily calories. I would avoid it like the plague.

ESSENTIAL CARBOHYDRATE?

Technically, there are no carbohydrates that we can't live without, meaning there are no essential carbohydrates. Carbs are energy-containing macronutrients that come in a simple form and a complex form. The simple carbs, or simple sugars, are glucose, fructose, and galactose. They often come in the form of disaccharides, which consist of two of these molecules. For example, table sugar, or sucrose, consists of fructose and glucose; and lactose in dairy consists of glucose and galactose. Simple carbs are rapidly absorbed, and very little digestion is needed to get them into the bloodstream.

Complex carbohydrates include starches and fiber. These are long chains of the simple sugars; they must be digested and broken down into smaller components to be absorbed. The body stores carbohydrates as long chains of glucose called glycogen. The muscles and liver store this glucose source for fueling muscle and brain function. However, the body doesn't need carbs for building glucose stores; it can do that by converting amino acids and fats into glucose.

It could be argued that fiber—long chains of carbohydrates that can't be absorbed—are critical for survival. They help the bacteria in the intestines produce essential nutrients and improve digestion. They may not be essential, but they need to be consumed as though they are.

When glucose is in short supply, such as when you're fasting or on a low-carb diet, enzymes in your body can convert amino acids to glucose. This ensures availability of glucose for brain function and other essential processes. Leucine is one of the only amino acids (lysine is the other) that cannot be converted to the sugar glucose (kryptonite). This makes leucine the anti-kryptonite.

Interestingly, even though leucine can't be converted to glucose in the body, it can be converted to ketones. This means that when sugars are sparse and adequate high-quality, leucine-rich proteins are available, leucine can become a source of the antioxidant, brain-supporting ketone pool. In essence, leucine can contribute to healthier metabolism and brain function. Even if you aren't ketogenic dieting, your body makes ketones after an overnight fast. This becomes an important way to fuel your brain and heart muscle during fasted cardio.

THE TOXICITY OF SUGAR

Consumed in large quantities, sugar is a very toxic substance. Rapidly absorbed sugars, such as simple sugars, cause very high levels of sugar in the blood. Excess sugar leads to "caramelization," or glycation of proteins, in a reaction called the Maillard reaction. This is the same reaction that turns bread brown when it's baked or toasted. The reaction releases free radicals that damage tissues and increase inflammation in the body.

This inflammation increases the risk of heart disease, cancer, and many other maladies. The body makes antioxidants that protect it from inflammation and free radical damage. The more these resources are drawn on to fight the damage of sugar, the less available they are for other tasks, such as helping you heal after exercise, aiding your recovery from stress, or protecting you against diseases.

Sugar is so toxic that the body makes insulin to rapidly clear the sugar from the bloodstream and push it into muscle and fat cells. An accumulation of sugar in the bloodstream causes the blood to become viscous, leading to large shifts in fluids and severe acidosis, which can be fatal. Diabetics whose disease is poorly controlled and who have elevated blood glucose levels end up with chronic problems, such as heart disease, kidney disease, loss of vision, nerve damage, and brain damage, that severely shorten their lifespan.

FRUCTOSE: SUGAR CALORIES AREN'T CREATED EQUAL

If sugar isn't available to disrupt your metabolism, your body runs more efficiently so that you store less calories and burn more fat. Even simple sugars vary in their effects on the body.

The dose determines the poison. —Paracelsus

Fructose is such a toxic substance that nature packages it tightly with fiber in the form of fruits to help limit its absorption. Fructose is the number one source of excess calories in America, mainly in the form of high fructose corn syrup (HFCS), which is pervasive in processed foods because it's so cheap to produce. Normal corn syrup is mostly glucose, but HFCS is corn syrup whose fructose content is between 42% and 55% of the total sugar content.

Because fructose doesn't immediately stimulate insulin release the way glucose does, it delays the decrease in appetite after a meal. In other words, fructose actually leaves you hungry longer, and thus you eat more. Fructose essentially tricks your body into gaining weight.

Excess fructose and other sugars are converted to triglycerides in the liver, leading to more stored fat. Fructose consumption can potentially cause more health problems than glucose. A study at UC Davis, in which subjects consumed 25% of their calories from glucose- or fructose-sweetened beverages for 10 weeks, showed significant disadvantages to fructose consumption. Those who drank the fructose beverage showed increased rates of conversion to fat and bad LDL cholesterol, decreased insulin sensitivity, and more abdominal fat deposits. Abdominal fat deposits generate more inflammation and further insulin resistance than the fat under the skin, leading to higher rates of metabolic syndrome, heart disease, and diabetes.

Metabolic Syndrome

- Increased abdominal fat
- Increased blood lipids
- Increased blood glucose
- Increased blood pressure
- Increased whole body inflammation

THE 1980s FAT-FREE FAD

President Dwight D. Eisenhower's heart attack in 1955 brought attention to cardiovascular disease. Dr. Ancel Keys began his *Seven Countries Study* to determine correlations between diet and heart disease. After years of examining various diets around the globe, he concluded that consumption of saturated fats led to elevated cholesterol and increased risk of heart disease. The study spurred significant policy changes that culminated in the fat-free food craze of the 1980s. Unfortunately, in retrospect, much of Dr. Keys' data was scientifically unsound.

The worst part of this story is that the changes made in the 1980s led to misconceptions and food manufacturing practices that actually increased the incidence of metabolic syndrome, diabetes, and heart disease in this country. To this day, many people believe that all fat is evil and that we should all eat fat-free foods.

Sad to say, the "calorie is a calorie" myth complicates the issue even further. The body doesn't treat the calories from fats, sugars, and proteins the same way. Protein is not as easily converted to fat as glucose is, and protein actually increases metabolism after consumption. Fat has more structural function (in cell membranes, the lining of nerves, hormones, etc.) than sugar. Fructose has very different effects on the body than glucose does. The body can make its own glucose, but it never makes fructose; it doesn't need fructose. Fructose is more easily converted to fat than any other macronutrient and is carried in the bloodstream as bad LDL cholesterol.

Food manufacturers used sugars and partially hydrogenated vegetable oils to make up for the palatability lost when they removed saturated fats from products. As it turned out, the added sugars led to higher triglyceride levels and increased risk of heart disease. Adding insult to injury, the partially hydrogenated vegetable oils, otherwise known as trans fat, cause severe inflammation and also increase the risk of heart disease.

The human body runs much more efficiently on fats than on glucose. Glucose metabolism leads to more damaging metabolites than the burning of fat or ketones. Many studies have shown that methods that increase fat and ketone use for energy, like intermittent fasting and a low-carbohydrate diet, improve body composition (decreased body fat, increased lean muscle) and reduce the risk of metabolic diseases like diabetes.

The Leucine Factor Diet focuses on eating healthier fats and less sugar, so you can enjoy better health and longevity. If I had realized how much sugar I was eating in yogurt, juice, and processed foods, I might have had less inflammation and less risk of the tendinitis that led to my bicep tendon rupture years ago. I learned that the best way to avoid sugar is to avoid processed foods. By eating a diet of whole foods from the periphery of the supermarket—where vegetables, healthy meats, dairy, and eggs are located—I created a physique that is healthy and lean with an award-winning six-pack.

6

THE LEUCINE FACTOR DIET PLAN

The scientifically based Leucine Factor Diet will help you achieve your goal, whether you want to lose weight, gain muscle, or just live healthy. To simplify your life, the Leucine Factor Diet phone app can guide you through the steps of personalizing the diet program for your goals and to maximize your leucine intake with each meal. You may find yourself fitting into one of the following three goal categories:

1. MAINTAIN HEALTH. You feel that you are at your ideal body weight and you want to maintain that weight while living healthy for longevity or between physique contests. Your focus is on balanced nutrition to support your desired level of activity. You may also like to take a holistic approach to longevity focusing on whole food nutrition and proper supplementation.

2. BUILD MUSCLE. You may want to build muscle for bodybuilding or performance—or you may just want to improve your strength. Muscle is metabolic currency, and this goal means you need more energy and fuel to build muscle. Gain as much muscle and strength as you want and fuel your competitive spirit.

3. GET LEAN. You want to lose extra fat weight while maintaining muscle. You may be preparing for a physique competition, you may need to make weight for a sport, or your doctor may have told you that you need to lose weight for health reasons. Losing weight means burning fat and sometimes, at the expense of losing some muscle. This diet will help you lose the fat and spare the muscle most effectively. There are no miracles here. The prescription for burning fat while keeping muscle is a proper diet and the right amount of exercise.

The Leucine Factor Diet is based on scientific principles that allow you to maximize lean muscle mass while losing fat or beefing up. The goal of any of the above categories is to stay anabolic and maintain your metabolic currency. Losing weight is largely a catabolic process, but anabolic stimuli can still help you to maintain muscle while losing fat. Believe it or not, you can actually burn fat *and* build muscle at the same time; however, the pounds might not come off the way you want them to. Muscle is more dense than fat, and building muscle keeps your weight up even when you burn fat. This diet helps you to maintain your muscle in the following ways:

Avoids the starvation response. The Leucine Factor Diet uses calculations or real-time biometric measurements of your daily calorie expenditure to make sure you are getting enough calories to reach your goal. If you are trying to burn fat, I recommend that most of your calorie deficit come from exercise rather than by limiting food. I recommend that you never restrict more than 250 calories from your diet and that your total energy deficit not initially exceed 500 calories (250 from food and 250 from exercise). Exceptions may apply in cases of health risks, when fat needs to come off faster. With an emphasis on healthy fats, protein, fibrous vegetables, and nutrient timing, you will feel fuller and less "starved" than on other more restrictive diet programs.

Optimizes protein intake. The American College of Sports Medicine and the American Dietetic Association recommend 0.8 grams of protein per pound of body weight per day for strength and endurance athletes, or nearly twice the amount of the recommended daily allowance. On the 5-MAD diet, this equates to 24 grams of protein per meal for a 150-pound man. Unfortunately, this is just not enough protein to supply the leucine needed for maximizing muscle growth or for maintaining health. In particular, as you will learn, it is not enough protein for optimizing leucine delivery. My personal experience and science support the use of substantially more protein to maximize muscle growth and prevent muscle breakdown in dieting. Sometimes you need to reduce your carbohydrate and fat intake to maximize fat burning. In such a case, you will go into starvation mode without the addition of protein for calories. Increasing the proportion of calories from protein increases metabolism and improves mobilization of fat stores. The Leucine Factor Diet includes no less than 1 gram of protein per pound of body weight per day. If you have any questions about the safety of this diet, consult your physician (see Safety of Protein Intake on page 37).

Provides optimal leucine at each meal. As you have already learned, leucine is an amazing amino acid. It signals your body to build muscle when adequate nutrients are present. Studies show that the leucine content of a protein affects its ability to boost muscle protein synthesis. Studies also support that leucine in a minimum quantity of 0.02 grams per pound of body weight per meal can maximize muscle protein synthesis.

One myth that comes up often is that your body can absorb only 20 to 30 grams of protein per meal. If this were true, it would be very hard to take in enough leucine to reach the 0.02 grams per pound of body weight per meal. This myth evolved from studies concluding that 20 grams of protein or essential amino acids maximized muscle protein synthesis. However, those studies did not evaluate the effect of consuming more protein on limiting muscle protein breakdown. Muscle protein is in constant flux between synthesis and breakdown. Physical activity tries to break it down, and the body has to build it up during rest and recovery. Consuming more protein will actually help limit muscle breakdown proportionately. So don't hold back because of incomplete science. Eat protein to build muscle *and* to limit it from breaking down.

MEETING LEUCINE NEEDS

In light of the leucine threshold to be reached with each meal, I recommend that you focus on the leucine content of your meals. Each food contains a different percentage of leucine. That's why I devised a metric called L-Factor points or "LFPs" that will help you recognize foods with enough leucine to meet your needs with each meal.

For number simplification, an LFP is 10 times the number of grams of leucine in 1 ounce of a food.

FOOD	AMOUNT OF LEUCINE	LFPs
Whole egg	0.3 grams	3 points
Turkey breast	0.5 grams	5 points
Wild salmon	0.6 grams	6 points
Romano cheese	0.9 grams	9 points

The Leucine Factor Diet applies points to each food based on the leucine content per ounce of that food. With each meal you need 0.20 points per pound of body weight. Thus, a 150-pound man needs 30 points per meal (150 x 0.20 = 30). For example, because 1 ounce of wild salmon has 6 points, the 150-pound man would have to eat 5 ounces of salmon (30 ÷ 6 = 5.0) to meet LFPs.

Science supports a minimum intake of approximately 20 LFPs per meal, with higher amounts leading to more muscle activation.

Maximizes antioxidant and micronutrient intake. With green leafy vegetables, the Leucine Factor Diet maximizes your intake of the vitamins and minerals you need to recover from workouts and the prebiotic fiber to boost the bugs in your belly (see Prebiotics/ Probiotics, page 108). The vitamins, minerals, and antioxidants from whole foods are very well absorbed. Vegetables are also rich in nitrates, which help to deliver valuable nitric oxide. Nitrates and the nitric oxide they produce improve performance, increase delivery of oxygen and nutrients to muscles, and help control blood pressure. I consider green fibrous and leafy vegetables to be a free food (see page 89).

Provides goal-oriented supplement advice. Nutritional supplements are essential to your success on the Leucine Factor Diet, unless you are a meticulous eater. When you aren't able to maximize your protein and leucine content through whole foods (especially when your calories are restricted or you don't have enough time to eat properly) supplements become a savior. A daily multivitamin ensures that you fulfill your micronutrient needs. Some supplements are essential to athletes and very active individuals. Supplements like creatine, beta-alanine, arginine/citrulline, and betaine boost strength and muscle endurance, leveling the playing field. Some supplements help increase metabolic rate and burn more fat throughout the day such, as black and cayenne pepper extracts.

FIGURE OUT YOUR LEUCINE FACTOR DIET

By following the steps below, you can create the best diet for attaining your goals. Adjust the diet weekly depending on your progress, attitude, energy level, and health. Sugars, desserts, and alcohol are not included in the Leucine Factor Diet. If you add these sweets or empty calories, you'll need to make up for it through added exercise or reductions in carbohydrate or fat calories in scheduled meals. If you decide to have a sugary, flavored latte instead of black coffee with Splenda, you will have to account for the calories in your next meal. Try to plan ahead even, with little cheats like this. If you know you have a latte every Tuesday morning, account for the carbs and fats in one or two of your meals that day.

The Five Steps to Your Leucine Factor Diet

I. Calculate your basal metabolic rate (BMR, page 81).

2. Calculate your activity factor (page 83).

3. Determine your total daily expenditure using your BMR and activity factor (page 84).

4. Calculate your macronutrient needs (page 85).

5. Create your Leucine Factor Diet (page 87).

Simplify the process of creating your Leucine Factor Diet plan; get the Leucine Factor phone app. Visit LeucineFactor.com for details.

CALCULATE YOUR BASAL METABOLIC RATE (BMR)

This calculation based on the equation below is the starting point for finding your total daily expenditure. The equation requires your height, goal weight, age, and sex. Notice that the calculation is made using your *goal weight* and not your current weight. More accurate assessments can be done if you know your body fat percentage (see the Katch-McArdle Formula on page 82).

> Your body fat percentage can be measured in a number of ways. The best way is to use skin fold calipers that can be purchased online (see LeucineFactor.com). You can easily learn how to do this by viewing videos online or by learning from a certified personal trainer familiar with the technique. Otherwise, some medical offices offer testing with machines like the Bod Pod or DEXA scanning. In addition to being expensive, this method can limit your ability to adjust your diet to your progress.

Harris-Benedict equation. As you begin performing calculations of your energy needs, please realize that equations for measuring your total daily expenditure can vary plus or minus 30% for individuals with the same body habitus. Our individual metabolic systems and the environments in which we live affect total daily expenditure and equations won't fit everyone's life and metabolism the same. These numbers are meant to be a starting point, and you should adjust your daily calories up or down each week if you aren't gaining or losing what you expect. Let's go through this equation for a 130-pound woman who is 35 years old, stands 5 feet 4 inches tall, has 20% body fat, and wants to be 120 pounds and leaner.

MEN:

BMR = 66 + (6.23 x goal weight in pounds) + (12.7 x height in inches) – (6.8 x age in years)

WOMEN:

BMR = 655 + (4.35 x goal weight in pounds) + (4.7 x height in inches) – (4.7 x age in years)

Our 35-year-old, 5-foot-4-inch (or 64-inch), 130-pound woman who wants to be 120 pounds:

BMR = 655 + (4.35 x 120) + (4.7 x 64) – (4.7 x 35) = 655 + 522 + 301 – 165 = 1313 calories per day

Katch-McArdle formula. You can use this formula if you know your lean mass from body fat percentage:

BMR = 370 + (9.8 x lean mass in pounds)

CALCULATION FOR LEAN MASS

Body fat percentage of total body weight = total fat weight

So if our hypothetical woman has 20% body fat, then 0.20 x 130 = 26 pounds of fat

Lean mass = total body weight – total fat weight

130 – 26 = 104 lean pounds

BMR = 370 + (9.8 x 104) = 1389 calories per day

Notice that the number of calories is higher than in the Harris-Benedict equation. If you have more lean mass, you will burn more calories in the day. Knowing your body fat percentage gives you a slightly more accurate reading than one based on norms for the general population.

However, I want you to focus on the fact that these numbers are just estimates and a starting point for your diet. The numbers have inherent problems because everyone's metabolism is different. You will adjust your diet as you go to match your goals.

For instance, if your goal is to lose 1 pound per week, and in the first week you lose only 0.5 pounds despite strictly following the diet, you know that over the course of a week you need to use up more calories through exercise or cut them through dietary changes. Because 3500 calories is approximately equivalent to 1 pound of fat, that means your 0.5-pound loss is equal to about 1750 calories. You need another reduction of 1750 calories to achieve the loss of a full pound. That translates to a reduction of 250 calories per day (1750 ÷ 7 = 250).

3500 calories burned = 1 pound of body fat burned

CALCULATE YOUR ACTIVITY FACTOR

After figuring out your BMR, you need to consider your level of activity to calculate your total daily energy expenditure (TDE). An activity monitor can help you measure your activity level; otherwise use standardized numbers (see the chart below).

ACTIVITY LEVEL	CALORIE CALCULATION
Sedentary (little or no exercise)	BMR x 1.2
Lightly Active (light exercise or sports 1–3 days a week)	BMR x 1.375
Moderately Active (moderate exercise or sports 3–5 days a week)	BMR x 1.55
Very Active (hard exercise or sports 6–7 days a week)	BMR x 1.725
Extra Active (very hard daily exercise or sports plus physical job or twice-a-day training)	BMR x 1.9

DETERMINE YOUR TOTAL DAILY EXPENDITURE (TDE)

Multiply your BMR by your activity factor to estimate the total calories you burn each day, or total daily expenditure (TDE). Now you need to adjust the TDE based on your goal. When setting up a goal, either use an activity factor or start with the activity level of a sedentary individual, 1.2.

TDE = BMR x 1.2

This gives you a baseline on which to add or subtract calories in the form of food or exercise.

Maintain Health. You can use an activity factor based on your actual level of activity to estimate calories expended through activity. As an alternative, start with the baseline of BMR x 1.2 and add the total estimated calories burned for all your activities in a day. Take the example of the 130-pound, 5-foot-4-inch woman with the BMR of 1313 (calculated with the Harris-Benedict equation). Her TDE would be 1576 if she were sedentary, and 1826 if she expended 250 calories through exercise.

1313 BMR x 1.2 = 1576 TDE

1576 TDE + 250 calories of exercise = 1826 TDE with exercise

This is our hypothetical woman's goal number of calories to consume when doing 250 calories of exercise per day. It will allow her to maintain her weight, without gaining or losing. Again, estimates of calorie expenditure based on activity factor or other measures (for example, activity monitors, cardio equipment calculations, or activity estimates) have inherent statistical errors, and you will need to adjust your diet according to your progress.

Remember, your body is unique and doesn't fit any one formula.

Build Muscle. I recommend that you add 250 calories to your TDE. This will ensure that you have plenty of calories to remain anabolic.

Note: If you add more than 250 extra calories, chances are that you will put on a little fat weight. If adding more than 250 calories is okay for your goal, try and add more calories from protein. Additional protein calories can add mass without affecting fat accumulation as much as additional carbohydrates would. Stick to high-quality, leucine-rich proteins like whey isolates.

Get Lean. I recommend cutting no more than 250 calories from your diet. As your deficit approaches more than 500 calories per day, you run the risk of significant muscle loss and a slowing of your basal metabolic rate leading to the starvation response. Slow and steady weight loss is always better than rapid weight loss (with only few exceptions, such as in morbid obesity and physique contest dieting).

If our hypothetical 130-pound, 5-foot-4-inch woman wanted to get lean through changes to her diet, she would cut 250 calories from her TDE of 1826 (the 1826 calories includes the added 250 calories from exercise; this could be assumed by an activity factor greater than sedentary rather than known calories if preferred):

1826 – 250 = 1576 calories from food

On a sedentary day, this woman's TDE would be 1576 and thus subtracting 250 calories from 1576 would be 1326 calories per day; I don't recommend a sedentary lifestyle.

CALCULATE YOUR MACRONUTRIENT NEEDS

Once you have calculated your total daily expenditure, including exercise, you can determine your macronutrient needs.

Your protein intake will be a minimum of 1 gram per pound of body weight, and enough to generate 0.20 L-Factor points per pound per meal (points calculations will come in later).

Subtract the number of calories obtained from 1 gram of protein per pound of body weight from your TDE. This is calculated as grams of protein x 4 calories per gram. Essentially this is the same as calculating:

TDE – (4 x goal body weight) = calories left after protein needs are met

For our hypothetical woman, the calculation works out as follows:

1576 – (4 x 120) = 1096 calories left after protein needs are met

After subtracting the protein calories, divide the remaining calories into fat and carbohydrate calories based on your goal category. Remember, fats provide 9 calories per gram, and carbohydrates provide 4 calories per gram.

Maintain Health. Divide the remaining calories 50/50 between carbs and fats.

Build Muscle. Allot 60% of the remaining calories to carbs and 40% to fats.

Get Lean. Allot 40% of the remaining calories to carbs and 60% to fats.

40% of 1096 calories = 438 calories as carbs ÷ 4 calories per gram = 110 grams of carbs per day

60% of 1096 calories = 658 calories as fat ÷ 9 calories per gram= 73 grams of fats per day

With the total grams of each macronutrient now calculated, divide each equally over five meals per day. If our hypothetical woman's goal is to get lean, here's how she divides her macronutrients:

120 grams of protein = 24 grams of protein per meal

110 grams of carbs = 22 grams of carbs per meal

73 grams of fats = 15 grams of fats per meal

CREATE YOUR LEUCINE FACTOR DIET

After determining your macronutrient requirements for each meal, select your favorite foods from the Leucine Factor Diet preferred foods list (see page 161).

Wild salmon has about 5.8 LFPs per ounce, turkey breast has about 5.3 LFPs per ounce, 85% ground beef has 6.1 LFPs per ounce.

Once you have selected your protein sources, you can determine if your leucine content for each meal is high enough. Remember, you need 0.20 LFPs per meal per pound of body weight. If a meal doesn't contain enough leucine, then you need to make adjustments to meet your needs or restrict excess fat or carbs.

Let's say our hypothetical woman whose goal weight is 120 pounds has chosen 85% ground beef. To get the LFPs she needs from 85% ground beef, she does the following calculations:

120 x .20 L-Factor points per pound = 24 L-Factor points per meal

For 85% ground beef: 24 LFPs ÷ 6.1 points per ounce = 3.9 ounces of 85% ground beef per meal

However, 85% ground beef contains 7.9 grams of protein per ounce, and 3.9 x 7.9 = approximately 31 grams of protein. That means the woman in our example will get 7 more grams of protein than she needs (31 – 24 = 7). In someone trying to get lean, we will remove the extra protein calories equally from carbohydrate. Thus, the carbohydrates allowed for this meal will drop by 7 grams as protein is the same calories per gram as carbohydrate (4 calories per gram); the problem usually comes in the form of excess fats. Also note that 85% ground beef has 4.3 grams of fat per ounce, and 3.9 x 4.3 = approximately 17 grams of fat. Since this exceeds her fat allotment by 2 grams, the extra calories would need to be cut from carbs further, or she should just choose a leaner cut of meat.

To make life simpler, when calculations are within plus or minus 5 grams of fat or carbohydrate goals, simply accept the discrepancy and make note of it. If you are consistently at plus 5 grams of extra carbs or fats and you gain weight, then adjust your intake downward the next week.

> You must reach your minimum LFPs in each of the five meals. It is best to divide fats and carbohydrates evenly among the meals, but this is less critical than dividing protein evenly. If you want a meal with a little more fat (for example, salmon instead of tilapia), then have less fat in another meal that day (for example, chicken breast instead of beef steak or egg white instead of whole egg).

Supplemental protein. If your body weight–based protein needs do not meet your L-Factor points for a given protein, you must add supplemental protein or leucine to meals. This can be done in the form of added dietary protein (chicken, fish, lean meats) or a supplement (whey, soy, casein, leucine chew, etc.).

Maintain health and get lean goals. If the added protein brings in extra fat calories, account for them by cutting an equal number of calories from carbohydrates.

Build muscle goal. Accept the extra protein and fat calories without any other changes.

Add supplemental leucine. Often, just adding 1 gram of leucine (10 LFPs) to your meal from a supplement will suffice if you are meeting your 1 gram of protein per pound of body weight requirement through high-quality, complete protein. A leucine pill will not count toward daily calories, but a bar or foods will count and you'll need to adjust your fat and carb totals.

THE EXTRAS

VEGETABLES: FREE FOODS!

In the Leucine Factor Diet, green leafy or stalked vegetable are a free food. You might argue that broccoli has nearly 2 grams of carbs per ounce and spinach 1 gram of carbs per ounce, but I don't care. We need more vegetables. They are the perfect combination of fiber, micronutrients like vitamins and minerals, and complex antioxidant compounds.

The carbohydrates found in nature come packaged with fiber. Look at sugar cane and wheat. They are very dense with fiber until they are processed into unhealthy, easily digested white sugar and flour. The carbohydrates in vegetables are typically more complex and much more slowly absorbed than those in fruits. Furthermore, the carbohydrate density is much less. Meaning, you can eat a lot more vegetables and get a satisfying full feeling without worrying about calories as you do with fruits.

The phytochemicals produced by vegetables are too numerous to review in this book. Green vegetables produce compounds that have antioxidant, anti-inflammatory, anti-cancer, and anti-toxin properties. It is important to note that although many supplement companies isolate these compounds for burning fat, building muscle, or staying healthy, the phytochemicals in vegetables work best when incorporated with the other nutrients that vegetables supply, including fiber.

I recommend eating some sort of green leafy or stalked vegetable with each of the five meals per day. Eating them raw or steamed is preferable, as one can be assured that their nutrients will be unaltered by processing. If you are supplementing with a ready-to-drink shake or a powder in one or two of the meals, then plan to carry a small bag of vegetables for a snack. Make some homemade kale chips or put broccoli florets in the freezer. Frozen vegetables will thaw out by the time you are ready to enjoy them. Blending vegetables into shakes works well as long as you don't strain out the fiber.

When you get your diet in alignment with essential amino acids and fatty acids, you become less dependent on grains for carbohydrate. You will start to notice the natural sweetness of many vegetables once you have cut your addiction to sugars and starches.

As for fruits, it is important to think of them as a luxury. Fruits need to fit into your carbohydrate consumption limits based on your goals. Bananas, apples, pears, kiwi, blueberries, raspberries, and many other fruits have nutritional value from phytochemicals, vitamins, and fiber, but the amount of simple carbohydrate can throw off your metabolism by spiking blood glucose levels and insulin. Especially avoid juicing fruits as they lose their bulk fiber value. Fruits are nature's candy: consider them a treat.

The Leucine Factor phone app can simplify this entire process of creating goal-oriented leucine-rich meals by linking the numbers directly to your foods and giving you per-meal quantities and LFPs. Using the app weekly will help you adjust your progress toward your goals.

SNACKS

You'll have to account for any additional snacks or treats by adjusting future meals or adding exercise. As you have learned, sugar is the enemy of success. Limit fruits and sugars to post-workout carbs or during intense training/competition sessions. Snacking should come in the form of tree nuts and fresh fibrous vegetables. However, it is best to avoid snacking and instead stick to the 5-MAD diet, which means meals every 3 hours.

If you break from the scheduled diet plan, get back on track with the next meal by not overeating and making sure that you achieve your L-Factor point goal. If you overeat carbs or fats in one meal, try to cut back a little on subsequent meals that day, but maintain protein intake to achieve your needed level of leucine.

CONDIMENTS

Use condiments in moderation—but pay attention to calories if you use them in larger amounts. If you want to use a salad dressing such as oil and vinegar, then include the oil in your fat calories. Mustard is better than ketchup, which often contains sugar, and mayo is rarely healthy. Spices—such as cayenne, cinnamon, nutmeg, garlic powder, pepper, and turmeric—are a great way to add flavor without calories. Occasionally, spices add some health benefit. For example, cinnamon improves blood glucose levels, turmeric reduces inflammation, and cayenne improves metabolic rate. Your food need not be bland. As you get more familiar with which foods fit your LFP needs, work on recipes that are in accordance with those needs. Salt your foods only if needed and in moderation. Since you will be focusing on natural, whole foods from the grocery store, sodium should not be a problem.

Sodium is typically not a problem in the Leucine Factor Diet as I encourage you to avoid processed foods. Shop in the periphery of the grocery store such as the produce section, meat counter, and dairy coolers. Salt your meals to taste and in moderation. Get creative with spices like cinnamon, turmeric, and oregano to limit your salt intake.

BEVERAGES

Sugar-free beverages such as water, coffee, Crystal Light, and artificially sweetened waters are allowed as much and as often as desired. Black coffee is encouraged for its antioxidant benefits and mind- and body-boosting caffeine. Stay hydrated with at least 8 ounces of water with or after each meal.

Artificial Sweeteners

I have to admit, I tend to use artificial sweeteners like Splenda and NutraSweet fairly regularly. I have a little Splenda in my black coffee or with cinnamon on my oatmeal nearly every day. I believe that these are safe compounds, in moderation, as the FDA states. However, the science of foods and medicine is constantly evolving, and it is important to watch for research that might change this position.

In my opinion, the health effects of sugars are much more harmful than those of artificial sweeteners. For instance, only 15% of Splenda is actually absorbed, and what is absorbed is secreted unchanged in the urine. NutraSweet is essentially two amino acids, aspartic acid and phenylalanine. The steviol glycosides in Stevia are naturally derived, but you may find them quite bitter.

Sugar alcohols used in artificial sweeteners, like mannitol, sorbitol, and erythritol, have fewer calories, don't raise blood glucose, and don't cause tooth decay; but some people get GI side effects from their laxative effects. Saccharin is the least "natural" of the artificial sweeteners; I don't recommend it.

As you wean off of carbohydrates and sugars in your diet, you will actually find that many foods are naturally sweet. If you need sweeteners, use them moderately. Limit diet soda consumption and try water with lemon or lime wedges for a hint of flavor.

NUTRIENT TIMING AND WORKOUTS

Time your meals so that a meal or shake follows within 1 hour of your workout session. If you are building muscle, have half of the meal before your workout session and the other half afterward. If you are trying to maintain health, you can have it either way; half before and half afterward or all of it afterward. If your goal is to get lean, have the meal post-workout, skipping carbs and distributing them evenly in other meals, or using their absence as part of your calorie deficit.

By delaying the intake of carbs after a workout, you continue the fat-burning potential of the workout for a few hours, but get your protein for the leucine!

SUPPLEMENTS

Even though the majority of your nutrition should come from whole unprocessed foods, nutritional supplements, especially vitamins and sports supplements, play a critical role in helping you reach your goals in sport and longevity. It can be very difficult to get all the nutrients you need to maximize health when you are living a hectic life of work, family, and exercise.

Essential Supplements

On a daily basis, everyone should take a multivitamin with minerals, 2 grams of fish oil, 2000 units of vitamin D (if not contained in the multivitamin), and a probiotic supplement.

Increases in activity or stress, or a combination of the two, can prompt a need for added nutrients that are difficult to get through regular meals. For instance, making sure you get your daily requirement of all essential vitamins and minerals by assessing the nutrient content of everything you eat is a daunting task! Taking a daily multivitamin with minerals relieves you of that job.

As another example, optimizing your recovery from exercise through leucine-rich foods can be a challenge when it comes to meeting your LFP requirement per meal. That's why I developed the leucine-rich L-Factor Bar. It will augment or even replace a meal. If your meal is 10 points short of your LFP requirement, eating one-third of an L-Factor Bar will help you meet your goal. Further, using a meal replacement shake for one or two of your meals in the day is a great way to get high-quality, leucine-rich whey protein that will meet your LFP goal.

There are thousands of supplements in the marketplace, and sorting through which ones are best for you and your goals can be very challenging. My objective is to simplify this selection process as much as possible by recommending supplements that are of the highest quality and have undergone rigorous scientific scrutiny.

When shopping for or using supplements, it is important to keep the following in mind:

1. CHOOSE SUPPLEMENTS THAT ADDRESS NUTRIENT DEFICIENCIES OR WORKOUT GOALS.

Deficiencies occur when a diet lacks important nutrients. For example, if you don't eat five servings of vegetables a day, you may lack essential vitamins, minerals, antioxidants, and fiber. In this case, you should consider a fiber supplement and a multivitamin. Similarly, you may find it difficult to eat five protein meals of lean meat, dairy, or eggs. Here, you would benefit from a protein/leucine supplement. If you are a vegetarian, you should consider creatine and soy protein supplementation because your diet will likely be deficient in those nutrients.

When your goal is to build or maintain as much muscle as possible, you will find that whey protein, creatine, HMB, and other performance-enhancing supplements are critical. Science supports that adding many of these supplements to a healthy diet will boost performance. It may not necessarily address an essential nutrient deficiency, but it may help you overcome a relative deficiency as hard training and dieting requires added nutrients. For example, studies show that when athletes in training are given either a placebo (sugar pill) or creatine, the creatine-supplemented athletes have greater strength, greater power output, and gains in lean mass. The strength athlete may not have been getting enough creatine from the meats in his diet.

2. AVOID TOO MUCH OF A GOOD THING. MORE ISN'T ALWAYS BETTER.

The "more is better" mentality is pervasive. Just as you can overtrain in the gym, you can "oversupplement." Taking 500 grams of protein every day in the form of a whey protein drink is not going to turn you into the Incredible Hulk. Your body takes the protein it needs for building muscle and repairing tissues, and uses the rest as energy or eliminates it through the kidneys. Excesses of protein to this extreme may even be detrimental and result in organ damage. Anything in excess, including water, is potentially risky.

The kind of stimulants found in fat-burning and pre-workout supplements can be especially dangerous when taken in excessive amounts. There are many case reports in the medical literature and media about the possible harm in excessive use of stimulant supplements. This is not to say that you can't use these supplements; you have to use them as directed and in a sensible manner. For instance, you shouldn't take fat burners so that you can spend a night on the town drinking alcohol. This can be a deadly combination.

3. NOT ALL SUPPLEMENTS WORK FOR EVERYONE. BE SCIENTIFIC AND FIGURE OUT WHAT WORKS FOR YOU.

I developed the Leucine Factor Diet from a scientific perspective, with the intention that you profit from the same perspective. It is very important that you choose your supplements based on scientific evidence that they actually work. You should choose supplements that have been studied in people similar to you and have proven effectiveness in your type of training goal.

For instance, if you are a well-trained sprinter, a study demonstrating that a supplement improves sprint speed in otherwise sedentary persons does not apply to you as much as it does to novice athletes. Novices often show incredible responses when introduced to training protocols and supplements. If you can't find any studies on athletes like you, then you may need to conduct your own experiment—even though this is basically a study in which you are the only subject. The results will be anecdotal to everyone else and specific to you.

Here's what to do: Choose a supplement that is intended to enhance your goal, whether that's to maintain health, build muscle, or get lean. Then take it as directed in conjunction with the Standardized Exercise Test, described on page 97. Record your performance before and after supplementation. Be specific and objective. If the supplement works, then bravo! If it doesn't work, then move on to the next supplement.

If you want to find studies on a particular supplement, search its name and the outcome you are interested in (for example, creatine and strength) at www.pubmed.gov. If you are a student, chances are that you have access to an online library where you can get articles of interest. While an undergrad, I would read about a supplement or training technique in a magazine, and I would look up the science in the library to find the scientific article it related to. By doing this, I became scientific about my training and familiarized myself with the scientific process, thus improving my ability to critically analyze new products on the market. Obviously, this may not be the best way for most. Follow my blog and my supplement performance column in *Muscular Development Magazine* for my analysis of new supplement ingredients in the market.

The Standardized Exercise Test

- Pick an exercise task that allows you to measure your goal after taking a supplement (for example, one rep max weight on bench press, or time to complete a 1-mile run).

- Before starting the supplement, pick the same time of day and arrange similar meals for the week via the Leucine Factor Diet, and be adequately rested from your previous exercise bouts.

- Keep a record of the time or weight achieved (or whatever the measure might be) in the baseline bout.

- After 2 to 4 weeks of training on the supplement, re-create the same conditions and perform your test again. That being said, some supplements are meant to have an immediate effect and can be tried and tested right after consuming. For instance, some pre-workout supplements say they can boost strength in the first use. In this case, do a workout without it, measure your task (for example, 1 rep max), rest well, and then try it again with the supplement after 1 week.

- When you compare two different supplements, try to re-create the same test, meal, and rest conditions.

4. BEWARE OF PROPRIETARY BLENDS AND ROGUE BRANDS.
A proprietary blend is a list of ingredients that the supplement company creates to keep the quantities of each ingredient a secret. Often, a label will contain a list of multiple extracts and supplements with a summary that says it contains X number of milligrams. Unfortunately, this leaves the door open for the manufacturer to perform the nefarious process of "pixie dusting." That is, it may put extremely small and ineffective quantities of some nutrients in the

blend while making the majority of the blend out of the cheapest nutrient. This can be counterproductive to your goals and a waste of your money.

Supplements aren't regulated by the U.S. Food and Drug Administration (FDA) in the same way as prescription drugs. Although the FDA sets production standards and the Federal Trade Commission (FTC) establishes rules for making claims, neither agency requires clinical trials to prove quality, safety, or effectiveness. Unfortunately, this often results in the marketing of supplements that can cause harm. When enough harm is done, the FDA gets wind of the problem and investigates. If action is warranted, the FDA can then remove the supplement from the market.

The FDA doesn't require pre-market testing of dietary supplements. However, under the law, manufacturers are responsible for making sure their products are safe before they go to market, and the claims on their labels must be accurate and truthful. The FDA has the responsibility to take action against any unsafe product that reaches the market. False and misleading claims made by supplement manufacturers can lead to legal action by the FDA, FTC, and consumers who feel misled.

Stick with brands that are known to have good production standards with regular testing of the quality and safety of their supplements, such as GNC Brand, AboutTime Protein, and The L-Factor Bar. There are many regulatory bodies that monitor the quality of supplement manufactures. Visit the blog at LeucineFactor.com for a list of these. Rogue brands that sell supplements with lofty claims pop up almost every day as do lawsuits against them for false advertising and physical harm. Supplements that refer to their effectiveness in relation to performance-enhancing drugs are particularly suspicious (for example, "just as effective as the steroid Anavar" or supplements with names similar to drugs, like Novadex or Ostarine). Don't buy into these fake and often unsafe snake oils.

5. CHECK WITH YOUR PHYSICIAN FIRST.

Dietary supplements do not come without risk. You are taking them to make up for a deficiency, enhance your performance, or improve your health. This means you are looking for an "effect." It almost goes without saying that anything that can have an effect on your body's physiology can have a side effect. That is, supplements and medications are not perfect and can have unintended or unexpected consequences.

It is important to research the supplements you are taking to understand possible side effects. This is especially a good idea for certain people. If you are pregnant, are nursing a baby, or have a chronic medical condition such as diabetes, high blood pressure, heart disease, thin blood, anemia, or anxiety or depression, be sure to consult your doctor before taking any supplement. Parents should check with their pediatrician before giving any supplements to their children. If you were prescribed a medication and heard that a supplement could replace it, ask your doctor if he or she agrees before you stop the medication. Supplements and herbal extracts often contain active ingredients with strong physiological effects that can interact with medications or medical conditions.

Taking supplements with medications (prescription or OTC drugs) could produce adverse effects. Although rare, the reaction of medication and supplements can result in life-threatening events. The most common examples are interactions with prescription blood thinners like warfarin: Ginkgo biloba (an herbal supplement for memory), aspirin, vitamin E, and fish oil can all thin the blood dangerously in combination with warfarin. Additionally, taking excessive vitamin K can impede the action of warfarin.

It is especially important to inform your surgeon of any supplement you are taking because many supplements affect healing or bleeding. Some of these supplements need to be stopped at least 2 to 3 weeks ahead of your procedure to avoid potentially dangerous outcomes. Take a list of your supplements to your doctor's appointment.

RECOMMENDED SUPPLEMENTS

Multivitamin with minerals. A multivitamin is probably the single most important supplement that all of us should take. Most Americans do not consume enough of their daily vitamin and mineral requirements from food. I am not saying that a multivitamin should replace a healthy diet, but sometimes we skimp on vegetables, which provide so many vitamins and minerals. To avoid deficiencies and their impact on health, performance, and recovery, take a multivitamin with minerals as part of your daily routine—it's safe and effective. According to studies, a multivitamin may even increase your longevity.

Whey protein. As discussed earlier, whey protein is a very special protein from a health and muscle growth perspective. Its high leucine content is thought to contribute to its superior ability to rebuild muscle through activation of muscle protein synthesis. Whey protein isolates and hydrolysates are particularly useful. Whey protein shakes and bars can be used as a snack to meet protein and leucine requirements throughout the day. Microfiltered whey isolate mixes well in oatmeal and smoothies.

Fish oil. Many studies suggest that fish oil is effective in improving cardiovascular health and longevity. It may even enhance recovery from exercise, and its anti-inflammatory effect can soothe sore joints. It's the omega-3 fatty acids in fish oil that are crucial for good health. To find out more about omega-3s and why it's important to improve your omega-3 to omega-6 ratio, see Essential Fats on page 62.

Fish oil is a source of the best omega-3 fatty acids for your health: DHA and EPA. Fish oil supplements or fatty fish like salmon are better sources of omega-3s than foods such as canola oil, soybeans, flax, walnuts, and algae. However, if your diet is high in saturated fats and omega-6 fatty acids, a fish oil supplement will have little effect in tipping the balance toward healthy omega-3s. Eat more grass-fed and free-range meats as well as fish and eggs to improve the omega-3 content of your meals. A dose of 2 grams per day of fish oil is most often recommended.

Creatine. This compound produced in the liver is also consumed in meat and as a supplement. We get about half of our creatine requirement from meat, so if you are a vegetarian you should take a creatine supplement. However, supplementation shouldn't be limited to vegetarians—it can be valuable for athletes generally.

The role of creatine in the body is to provide an immediate source of energy. All muscle action is powered by a compound called adenosine triphosphate (ATP). Creatine's job is to restore ATP rapidly when it is consumed by the muscle for contraction.

Perhaps the best performance-enhancing supplement available to the strength athlete, creatine's use and safety for a variety of sports and training conditions is supported by scientific literature. If you want to build muscle or become stronger and you aren't familiar with the beneficial effects of creatine, you are a step behind your competition.

Creatine has been a game changer in sports nutrition and is found in an extraordinary number of sports supplements. With all the supplement gimmicks out there, creatine has proved many times over that it is the real deal in building muscle and improving sports performance. A vast field of research explains just how creatine supplementation improves performance. It was initially thought that creatine would be useful only in buffering short bursts of energy, but recent research has demonstrated how it can improve endurance by increasing blood volume, glycogen storage, and respiratory efficiency.

Of importance to Leucine Factor dieters is creatine's ability to improve muscle mass. In fact, supplementation with creatine, protein, and carbohydrate seems to be ideal for muscle growth. In one study, creatine induced a greater than 20% increase in a muscle growth factor and a 100% increase in lean body mass. More recent studies have demonstrated an added antioxidant and DNA protective effect of creatine supplementation, which presumably could improve recovery from intense exercise and dieting.

Research Update

Myostatin is a protein that inhibits muscle growth. Laboratory data now suggests that the amino acid leucine, its metabolite HMB, and creatine are all capable of counteracting the actions of myostatin. These three are the coveted "myostatin inhibitors."

It should be said that not everyone responds to creatine use. You are more likely to respond if you have lower initial muscle creatine stores (vegetarians), if you have a greater quantity of fast-twitch muscle, or if you are a first-time creatine user.

A number of studies have shown the relative safety of creatine supplementation in young and even elderly adults. The common misconception that creatine is unsafe for the kidneys has not been proven in the scientific literature. Although creatine appears to be safe for children and adolescents, the International Society of Sports Nutrition has suggested restricting use to competitive athletes who are post-puberty, eat a well-balanced diet, and are under the supervision of parents and qualified professionals. Furthermore, it recommends using high-quality products at only the recommended dosage.

In recent years, various types of creatine have come on the market, especially salts and esters. Creatine salts such as pyruvate and citrate forms may be slightly better absorbed, and the potential advantage of a salt like Kre-Alkalyn may be better digestive tolerability and better solubility in performance drinks. However, there is very little data to suggest that they have any benefit over the gold standard, creatine monohydrate, which has worked best for me. Given the lack of regulation, production oversight, and quality testing, some of these creatine derivatives may be harmful if not obtained from trustworthy companies.

Another form of creatine that is worth mentioning is polyethylene glycosylated creatine, or PEG-creatine, which has enhanced absorption because of the polyethylene glycol (PEG). It can be taken at a dose one-fourth of that used for creatine monohydrate and still produce improvement in muscular strength. In studies, subjects taking PEG-creatine did not gain weight like those taking creatine monohydrate despite similar increases in strength. This could be of benefit for sports with weight classes or when the goal is to lose weight.

Creatine is often taken in doses of 20 grams per day (four doses of 5 grams) for 5 to 7 days and then maintained at 5 to 10 grams per day afterward. It is well absorbed as part of a post-workout meal or shake. Creatine can be safely taken continuously. You do not have to cycle on and off creatine, even if your buddies at the gym swear it's true (a phenomenon called "broscience"). If you are involved in a sport that requires making weight, creatine monohydrate may cause some water retention, so you may want to stop supplementation a week or so before your weigh-ins.

In summary, creatine has revolutionized the supplement industry. The combination of creatine, carbohydrate, and protein is an essential component of any muscle-building routine. Creatine monohydrate is the gold standard, but other forms of creatine have their place in the market, especially PEG-creatine. Perhaps most important, creatine supplementation is safe and very effective.

Caffeine. Up to 90% of adults consume caffeine on a daily basis. Caffeine is quite possibly the most widely used drug in the world. With the ability to abolish fatigue and increase wakefulness, caffeine makes the world go 'round. If caffeine were to go into shortage, it could become more valuable than gold and global markets might crash from the lack of productivity. Everyone from truck drivers and airline pilots to soldiers and even surgeons get by on caffeine at some point.

Caffeine is heavily used in sports nutrition products intended for fat loss and workout enhancement. Numerous studies suggest that caffeine can improve sports performance, endurance, and recovery. It is so effective that it was once banned by the World Anti-Doping Agency for use in competitions like the Olympics. At a dose of 3 to 9 milligrams per kilogram of body weight, caffeine has a stimulating effect on the central nervous system: It improves focus and reduces perceived exertion (you can work harder but feel as though it takes the same effort).

To put this into perspective, 3 milligrams per kilogram of body weight of caffeine equals approximately two regular-size cups of coffee (approximately 16 ounces); and 9 milligrams per kilogram of body weight equals about five to six cups of coffee.

Coffee and Energy Drinks

Coffee supplies caffeine to keep humans productive. Nearly 500 billion cups of coffee are consumed each year worldwide. Coffee is the second largest traded commodity after oil, and nearly 40% of that coffee is produced in Brazil and Colombia. Coffee comes from a woody perennial tree that grows in high altitudes and comes in many species including Arabica and Robusta. Approximately three-quarters of all coffee beans produced are Arabica, but Robusta coffee is popular for its higher caffeine content.

Since coffee lives in a harsh, high-altitude environment, it requires defense mechanisms to survive. As a result, coffee is antioxidant-rich. Antioxidants impart health benefits by defending the body from the hazardous effects of free radicals. There are many conditions, ranging from cancers to diabetes, that antioxidants have been shown to benefit. Still, debate persists in the medical literature about whether coffee is beneficial or detrimental to human health. The safety limits of caffeine have traditionally been that healthy adults limit their intake to approximately 450 milligrams per day, although 600 milligrams per day may be an acceptable upper limit.

If you are looking for a natural boost to your pre-workout regimen, a 16-ounce cup of coffee may be all you need to increase focus, decrease perceived exertion, and protect you from free-radical oxidative damage. Hopefully, this means you train better, harder, and longer with improved recovery. Give it a try if you work out earlier in the day.

If coffee isn't for you, try energy drinks, which are among the most popular forms of caffeine. They contain caffeine mixed with some herbals and/or amino acid–like compounds such as taurine. These drinks have become increasingly popular, with more than 50% of college students drinking them on a regular basis. They go beyond the caffeine content of a Classic Coke, which contains 34 milligrams of caffeine per 12 ounces.

PRODUCT	CAFFEINE	CAFFEINE/OUNCE
Classic Coke (12 oz.)	34 milligrams	(2.83 mg/oz)
Red Bull (8 oz.)	80 milligrams	(10 mg/oz)
Monster Energy (16 oz.)	160 milligrams	(10 mg/oz)
Starbucks Grande Coffee (16 oz.)	330 milligrams	(20.62 mg/oz)
5-Hour Energy (2 oz.)	138 milligrams	(69 mg/oz)

In addition to performance-enhancing effects on endurance exercise, caffeine has been shown to increase performance in 60- to 180-second sprints and high-intensity intermittent exercise. Science suggests that caffeine's effects on the central nervous system may play a significant role here. The arousal effect and even a slight blunting of pain perception that comes with caffeine may explain the ability to push harder in short-duration activities (for example, maximal exertion in lifting or sprinting). I recommend keeping your doses around 200 to 400 milligrams per day as a pre-workout booster. This could be from drinking a 16-ounce coffee or from a pre-workout supplement containing caffeine. Coffee has healthy effects in itself that could be beneficial to your health and longevity with polyphenol antioxidants.

I caution you to keep your consumption on the lower end until you get used to that much caffeine. I also recommend doses on the lower end later in the afternoon. Consuming caffeine after 5 p.m. may disrupt your ability to fall asleep. Definitely avoid doses greater than 600 milligrams per day because of the risk of toxic effects. When consuming close to 600 milligrams of caffeine per day, be sure to divide it into two or three servings throughout the day. When taking any new supplements containing caffeine, conduct a tolerance test. That is, try taking one-half or less of the serving on your first try to test for any adverse reactions. If you tolerate the partial dose, slowly increase it until you get the desired effect.

Arginine and citrulline. The amino acid arginine is a building block for proteins. It is also used in the synthesis of nitric oxide, which is very important in many physiological processes, especially in improving blood flow. Furthermore, citrulline is a precursor to arginine, and nitrates in green vegetables and beetroot are excellent sources of nitric oxide.

Arginine and citrulline are often found in pre-workout supplements that are purported to boost nitric oxide and generate a "pump" by bringing more blood flow and nutrients to the muscle. They can improve performance by reducing neuromuscular fatigue and potentially enhance the anabolic response to exercise. Arginine boosts collagen synthesis, improves wound healing, and increases immune system function. It is especially useful in recovery from wounds and injury, for example, after surgery.

The typical dose of arginine for supplementation is 5 grams per day and citrulline 3 grams per day.

Polyphenol antioxidants. Antioxidants have effects that are very useful in recovery from exercise, especially after intense sessions that produce a lot of free radicals. Although free radicals play a role in stimulating adaptations to exercise in muscle and mitochondria, excessive free radicals cause significant tissue damage that can make recovery more difficult with prolonged soreness and weakness. Polyphenol antioxidants are found in many of the foods that we just don't eat enough of: vegetables.

A polyphenol antioxidant is a type of antioxidant containing a polyphenolic, or natural phenol structure. Plants make these compounds as a natural defense against the environment. For instance, grapes used in wine making are exposed to nature in environments that require great defenses against free radicals. Thus, they produce polyphenols like resveratrol (found in the skin of red grapes) as a defense mechanism to boost their own longevity resisting damage from excess sunlight or microorganisms. Recent studies suggest that resveratrol can activate anti-aging proteins called sirtuins and limit telomere shortening (see How the Environment Affects Genes, page 43) thought to lead to tissue aging.

Excessive oxidative stress and inflammation can reduce performance and lead to fatigue after exercise. If you are training with any level of intensity, you will likely produce excessive inflammation and oxidative stress. Using antioxidants in moderation may help with exercise recovery and relieve muscle soreness.

Melatonin. This natural hormone released by the pineal gland in the brain helps regulate sleep-wake cycles (circadian rhythms) by transmitting information about light and dark to the body. Its effects are numerous and span the spectrum of antioxidant, anti-cancer, anabolic, and immune effects. Melatonin can help you fall asleep and improve the restorative effects of sleep. It is usually taken at doses of 1 to 5 milligrams. Melatonin can even be effective for jet lag if taken on the day of departure at the time you would go to bed at your destination and for the following few days before bed.

Vitamin D$_3$. As will be discussed in Vitamin D and the Leucine Factor Diet (page 111), vitamin D is really a hormone made from cholesterol when sunlight hits your skin. It regulates the growth and development of many different types of cells, including muscle cells.

A vitamin D deficiency can cause significant muscle dysfunction and atrophy. Estimates of the prevalence of low vitamin D levels in American youth have ranged from 1% to 80%. Factors such as older age, higher body mass index, race/ethnicity, and hyperparathyroidism are associated with lower vitamin D concentrations in the blood. Levels tend to be more than 25% lower in winter, when days are shorter, than they are in summer. The next time you are at your doctor's office, ask for a vitamin D level as part of your lab testing.

Many people are vitamin D deficient despite self-proclaimed healthy eating. Because vitamin D is crucial for bones, muscles, and metabolism, I suggest supplementation of at least 2000 units to 4000 units per day.

Probiotics/prebiotics. Each of us carries more bacteria in our gastrointestinal (GI) tract than the number of people on the planet or the cells in the human body! The metabolic activity of the more than 500 species of organisms in your gut is nearly equal to that of any vital organ. In fact, the bacteria in your gut should be treated like another organ system. They support the tissues of the immune system, 80% of which is found in the GI tract.

The relationship between the microorganisms in your gut and the human body is symbiotic. This means that they cannot survive without you, and you cannot survive without them. Disruption of your gut flora can lead to severe disease and even death. The bacteria in your intestines perform many functions: strengthening the immune system, consuming unused energy substrates (like lactose), producing vitamins and hormones, and protecting against pathological species of bacteria. Research has shown that your healthy species of symbiotic bacteria produce compounds that are absorbed into your body, affecting your physiology and risk for disease in remarkable ways.

The science behind intestinal microorganisms is in its infancy and I expect great advances in the not-so-distant future. In the meantime, I recommend probiotic and prebiotic supplements to improve the microbiology of your gut.

Taking probiotic supplements with viable health-promoting microorganisms can improve digestion, the immune system, and even sports performance. Greek yogurt and fermented foods are useful in boosting healthy microorganisms, but they supply limited concentrations of the microorganisms compared with supplements. Recent research suggests that probiotic supplements block pathogens from penetrating the intestinal barrier after excessive high-intensity exercise. Symptoms such as bloating, cramping, and nausea after exercise may indicate a problem with the intestinal barrier—and the need for probiotic supplementation.

Prebiotics are essentially food for your gut bacteria. The most important prebiotic is fiber from your diet. Prebiotic supplements are those that promote healthy probiotic microorganism growth; these include fiber supplements and glutamine.

Fiber, an essential carbohydrate? Fiber is a type of carbohydrate that the body doesn't digest into sugars for energy production. Therefore, we don't typically consider fiber a caloric component of our meals or even think of it as "carbs." There are two types of fiber: soluble and insoluble. Soluble fiber is considered a prebiotic, which means it can be fermented by gut bacteria for fuel and thus contributes to a healthy GI tract. Insoluble fiber is more of a bulking agent without much of a prebiotic effect.

Both types of fiber impart health benefits. Some compounds produced during the fermentation of soluble fiber have important health functions, and insoluble fiber improves stool bulk and elimination to make you "regular." Sometimes the added bulk can be a disadvantage if you are dehydrated because constipation with uncomfortable bloating and gas can occur.

Fiber supplements are marketed to treat irregular bowel movements, lower cholesterol, reduce the risk of colon cancer, promote weight loss, and limit type 2 diabetes. Soluble fiber may be beneficial for treating constipation and abdominal discomfort from irritable bowel syndrome. The prebiotic function of soluble fiber may also promote healthy gut bacteria that relieve symptoms of inflammatory bowel diseases like Crohn's disease and ulcerative colitis.

Just the act of acknowledging the fiber content of foods may improve your diet significantly. High-fiber foods tend to be wholesome and natural. Whole foods take a little more time to eat and involve more mechanical digestion by the gut. In addition to making you eat more slowly, fiber in your diet may increase the time a food is in the upper GI tract and thus slows the appearance of glucose in your blood. Additionally, dietary fiber interacts with digestive enzymes causing less carbohydrate to be broken down to glucose for absorption. Diets rich in dietary fiber often are less energy dense—that is, they have fewer calories. So you tend to feel fuller on a high-fiber diet and won't consume as many calories as on a diet containing more processed, high-calorie foods.

Consistent intake of soluble fiber in foods like antioxidant-rich berries, vegetables, whole grains, and nuts is well known to reduce risk of the all-too-common diseases: obesity, diabetes, high cholesterol, cardiovascular disease, and many gastrointestinal disorders including constipation, inflammatory bowel disease, ulcerative colitis, hemorrhoids, Crohn's disease, diverticulitis, and colon cancer. All of the these disorders of the intestinal tract may benefit from the consumption of soluble fiber.

If reducing the risk of disease weren't enough, fiber may also help you live longer. A study of nearly 400,000 adults aged 50 to 71 found that those who consumed the most fiber were greater than 20% less likely to die of heart attack over the 9-year period of the study. In addition to the reduction in risk of death from heart disease, high-fiber diets correlated with lower rates of infections and cancer.

The average American's daily intake of dietary fiber—approximately 15 grams of fiber per day—is well below the 30 grams per day recommended by the major dietary governing bodies, including the American Dietetic Association. This lack of dietary fiber is likely due to the inundation of processed foods and too few vegetables consumed.

One aspect of dietary fiber that is often overlooked is calories. In the United States, food labeling includes soluble fiber, at 4 calories per gram, in the carbohydrate content of foods. However, studies suggest that because fiber is not well digested or absorbed, the calorie count may be closer to 2 calories per gram. This is why I don't usually include the carbohydrate content of green leafy vegetables in my calculations of macronutrient needs. I consider broccoli, asparagus, spinach, Brussels sprouts, and lettuce to be free foods.

VITAMIN D AND THE LEUCINE FACTOR DIET

It is fairly well known that Vitamin D plays a significant role in maintaining the health of bones and preventing the disease rickets. As important as having healthy bones is, the Leucine Factor Diet is all about maintaining and building lean muscle, strength, and longevity. So why does vitamin D get its own section? Well, as you will soon learn, vitamin D is a very special compound that acts more as a hormone than a vitamin. Its many functions go beyond bone health, and that means it deserves a bit of attention.

POWER OF THE SUN REVISITED

In The OJ Conundrum (page 13), I wrote about how manufacturers and their marketing firms try to make orange juice seem like bottled energy from the sun essential to your health. That just isn't true. OJ is just a tall glass of the strength- and health-robbing compound known as sugar. I called sugar the kryptonite that steals our strength and longevity.

Superman gained his strength from our yellow sun. How this occurred physiologically we may never know (thank you for the mystery, DC Comics). However, in our skin we make strength-giving vitamin D from ultraviolet sunlight and cholesterol.

Cholesterol → 7-dehydrocholesterol → Skin UV radiation exposure → Vitamin D$_3$

It is important to understand the importance of cholesterol in the human body. Cholesterol is known almost exclusively as a bad compound that you should limit in your diet for fear of heart disease. The fats that the body produces from ingested sugars are packaged with cholesterol and various proteins in the blood. It is this combination of packaged cholesterol and triglycerides that is bad for health. So, the fat-free fad that vilified saturated fats also gave cholesterol a bad name despite its many positive roles in health.

> HDL cholesterol or "good" cholesterol is cholesterol packaged with high-density lipoproteins. It helps carry cholesterol deposits away from the insides of your arteries. LDL cholesterol is the "bad" cholesterol" that is thought to contribute to greater risk of cardiovascular disease when elevated in the blood. In your blood work, high HDL is good and high LDL is bad for your health.

Cholesterol is important in the structure of cells and the synthesis of hormones. It provides the chemical backbone for many of the hormones that are called "steroid" hormones, including anabolic hormones like testosterone and catabolic hormones such as cortisol. Vitamin D can be considered a steroid-like hormone. Knowing the extensive function of vitamin D in the body, I'd rather consider it a hormone that we need to regulate than a vitamin we need a minimum amount of in our diets.

Vitamin D has a structure very similar to other steroid hormones and even acts similarly in tissues. Just like testosterone, vitamin D is carried in the blood on a transport protein. It is then passed into cells to act on a receptor that is in the same family as the steroid and thyroid hormone receptors. This receptor is able to turn on genes in the nucleus of many different types of cells throughout your body. Not only is vitamin D important for bones, but it also has receptors in tissues like the brain, muscles, heart, and immune system. Therefore, vitamin D is critical to the health of many organ systems and to longevity.

VITAMIN D AND THE ANTI-KRYPTONITE

Vitamin D has essential roles in the structure and function of the musculoskeletal system. A deficiency impairs bone growth and strength. Vitamin D levels in the blood have also been correlated to muscle cell contraction ability, muscle strength, and postural stability.

Although it is common knowledge that vitamin D is good for our bones by enhancing calcium absorption, it is less known that vitamin D is also good for muscles. This is most evident among the elderly. Low levels of vitamin D are associated with muscle weakness and fall risk as we age. In the elderly, it appears that there is a correlation between vitamin D levels and muscle mass. A low vitamin D level puts a person at a higher risk of falling. With weaker muscles come weaker bones and thus a higher risk of breaking those bones. The risk of death in an octogenarian who falls and sustains a hip fracture is up to 50% within a year of the fall.

We know from extensive research that we need more leucine in a meal to turn on muscle protein synthesis as we age. Studies also show that we need vitamin D to turn on our muscles' sensitivity to leucine and insulin. Aging decreases the sensitivity of muscle to the muscle-building effects of leucine and insulin. We also know that we tend to be more deficient in vitamin D as we age.

A great deal of research has focused on the health-promoting effects of vitamin D, especially with aging. Vitamin D intake up to 4000 units per day limits falls in the elderly and improves strength and balance. Surprisingly, vitamin D also lowers the rate of musculoskeletal injuries in otherwise healthy young dancers. Since dancers and the elderly rarely get time in the sun, it is important that their diets have rich sources of vitamin D.

SOURCES OF VITAMIN D

Vitamin D can be supplemented or consumed in foods that naturally contain it or are fortified with it. The vitamin D_3 form is the ideal supplement as it is presumed to be more biologically active because it is the form that your skin makes. Fatty fish species like catfish, salmon, and tuna are rich sources of vitamin D and leucine. Vitamin D is also found as vitamin D_2 form in mushrooms cultivated with exposure to UV light. However, there is controversy over whether the D_2 form is as active in your body as the D_3 form.

It is very important to get a vitamin D level with your blood work. Some people have a difficult time producing, absorbing, or storing vitamin D in their bodies and thus have extremely low levels. These individuals may need to consider high-dose supplementation with physician monitoring. I recommend that you consume 2000 to 4000 units of supplemental vitamin D_3 per day to maximize its function in your body. The Geriatric Society recommends a total of 4000 units of vitamin D from all sources per day. High doses in the 10,000 to 50,000 units range are not recommended without physician supervision.

7

BUILDING YOUR MEAL PLAN

I would guess that most readers of *The Leucine Factor Diet* are interested in getting lean. Maintaining muscle and burning fat is the essence of a leucine-optimized diet. Making sure that your diet contains optimal leucine in up to five satisfying meals per day is critical to maintaining muscle as metabolic currency, especially when consuming less calories than you are burning as when cutting fat to get lean.

It is very difficult to burn fat if the number of calories you take in is not at least slightly less than the number you expend. This is why a 250-calorie deficit is built into the "get lean" diet plan. You can add to the deficit through exercise, increased daily activity (for example, standing more often, taking the stairs instead of an elevator, parking farther from entrances), or metabolism boosters like capsaicin and supplements containing caffeine supplements.

Once you have calculated the number of calories per meal and your macronutrient breakdown of protein, fats, and carbs, it is time to create meals and stick to an exercise plan. In this chapter are my tips on how to create healthy meals and exercise in a way conducive to your time and goals. For a few of my favorite recipes, turn to the next chapter, starting on page 141.

MEAL PREPARATION

Making meals in advance is the best way to avoid the temptation to eat outside of your plan or stray from it. I always prepare my breakfasts and lunches for the weekdays on Sunday afternoon. Plastic storage containers are your friends. Invest in an insulated lunch bag that can hold a couple of meals with a cold pack. Further, have some protein powder ready in shaker cups or protein bars available for snacks.

Back in my bachelor days, I would use the microwave to cook all my food: tilapia, yams, egg whites, rice, oatmeal. Although microwaving is fast and easy, microwaved meals often lack creativity and flavor. That's why I like to use both the microwave and the oven/broiler to prepare meals. Steaming vegetables in the microwave while your fish or meat is cooking in the oven will save you time in the kitchen— and you'll end up with a tastier meal.

All Leucine Factor dieters should consider a daily multivitamin with minerals and whey protein supplementation. Maintain muscle as you age with the use of creatine and HMB supplements.

Drink plenty of water and avoid sugar. If you have sugar in your diet, it should come in the form of a fibrous fruit to help slow absorption and carry it out of your body. Avoid excessive saturated fats and focus on healthy polyunsaturated and monounsaturated fats that come in healthy fish oil and nuts.

BREAKFAST

Whether you make breakfast depends on your time in the morning and urgency to leave the house. Mixing whey protein like AboutTime Cinnamon Swirl with oatmeal or Greek yogurt is a quick way to get plenty of leucine. Easy-to-mix protein powders can help to flavor egg whites as well. Egg white whisked up like a meringue flavored with a fruity whey protein can be a yummy treat.

Egg white pancakes are a quick-and-easy breakfast that will keep in the refrigerator for 4 to 5 days. You can mix in oatmeal or egg yolks, depending on your fat and carbohydrate needs. Or instead of adding yolks, you can slather the pancakes with natural almond butter or peanut butter to get some healthy monounsaturated fats.

I like to make small vegetable and low-fat cheese omelets that can be stored in the refrigerator. An omelet is a great way to add variety as well as fiber and phytonutrients from green vegetables to your diet. Cheeses add a lot of leucine in small amounts with the ability to buy fat-free or low-fat to avoid exceeding your fat and calorie needs (1 ounce of cheese can be up to 10 L-Factor points). Vegetables like broccoli and asparagus have fiber for more complete digestion and removal of dietary cholesterol from the body.

LUNCH

For weekday lunches, I often cook a couple of large yams with about 2½ pounds of salmon, trout, or tilapia in the oven. After I evenly divide the cooked fish and yams into five meals, I put some frozen broccoli florets in my food storage containers. When I heat the meals at work, the florets warm up with the fish and yams. If you cook the fish well and refrigerate the meals, they will last the week.

Another option for preparing lunches or other midday meals is to cook them with your dinners during the week by doubling up on your cooking. Next day's lunch or midday meals can be leftovers.

Your dinners should have a very similar protein makeup as your lunches, or any other meals for that matter.

> The protein quantities should always be similar because you are trying to optimize your leucine intake. Fats and carbohydrates can vary from meal to meal as long as you don't exceed your needs for the day. Again, it is best to avoid overeating fats or carbs at any one meal as your body can process only so much at one time without storing the extra calories as fat.

DINNER

Dinner is a time when I tend to get a little more creative with meals. I'll try new recipes for seasoning meats, fish, poultry, or pork loin. Mashed cauliflower or spaghetti squash makes a great alternative to the usual potatoes, rice, or pasta. If I make pasta, it is often whole grain or gluten-free. I don't make any cream sauces, and I flavor pastas and vegetables with a little truffle oil when I need healthy fats. A salad of spinach, romaine, and kale can be a great replacement for carbs in the evening meal.

If I eat out during the week, often I'll order an extra chicken breast, another yam, or more rice to take home for a future meal. At most restaurants, you can ask the chef to make meals to your specifications. The kitchen can always steam a vegetable or grill meat without additives, butter, oils, or salt. However, ask if their meats have been marinated. If so, you may want to frequent another restaurant. Be careful with cheeses when you eat out. Most restaurants use more palatable fatty cheeses rather than the desired low-fat cheeses. Be sure to ask about the cheese in an entrée if it's not fully described.

When you embark on the Leucine Factor Diet, you may need to measure or weigh your cooked foods for a while to get a sense of what 6 ounces of grilled chicken or 8 ounces of salmon looks like. Soon you will learn to recognize the size of meat and fish servings that meet your leucine needs.

The bigger challenge comes in low-end fast food restaurants. Try to stick with salads containing chicken breast meat. Avoid croutons, extra fatty cheese, bacon bits, and heavy creamy or sweetened dressings. Replace these salad toppings with a squeeze of lemon or a teaspoon of oil with cider vinegar. For other dressings, ask for them on the side, and dip the tip of your fork in the dressing before lifting the lettuce with the fork. In the worst-case scenario, ordering a burger, discarding the bun, and dining on the patty with a salad can help you feel less guilty about eating at a fast food joint. For a beverage, choose unsweetened iced tea, water, or the occasional diet soda. I am a fan of avoiding end-of-the-day carbs and even early-morning carbs as this gives my body a good 12 hours to use fats for fuel. The fat-burning potential of my morning cardio is a little boosted, given that my last carbs were at 5 p.m. post-workout the day before. My next carbs will be with my breakfast after morning cardio, or sometimes I'll wait until my second meal and let the fat-burning machinery keep working.

"TWEENER" MEALS

Since this diet plan suggests five meals a day, you need to think about including a meal before a typical lunch and another between lunch and dinner. In reality, you should shoot for a meal every 3 hours. In doing so, you assure regular delivery of leucine. I like to have three or four whole food meals and one or two shakes or bars. My mid- to late-afternoon meals tend to be post-workout whey protein shakes with natural peanut butter and oats. My midmorning meal may be a shake, bar, more breakfast, or a meal of fish and a vegetable. These meals just need to meet you leucine and other macronutrient needs.

SAMPLE DIET AND EXERCISE PLANS

The diet and exercise plan you choose depends on your goal. I've provided sample plans for the following goals: 1) maintain health, 2) build muscle, and 3) get lean. Each of the sample plans is for a hypothetical person, but in each case let's pretend it's your plan. The Leucine Factor phone app will simplify the process of creating your diet plan.

MAINTAIN HEALTH

This diet plan is designed for people who feel they have attained their goal of a healthy body weight and adequate lean muscle. They want to maintain performance or health without any particular desire to build more muscle or lose weight. Having five whole food–based meals or having three whole food–based meals with protein bars or supplements in between works here. As with the other diet plans, space your meals (or meals and protein bars or supplements) every 3 hours or so, and time one of them to occur after your workout.

With this plan, you have to adjust your diet just as much as if you were dieting to get lean or build muscle. If you find that you are not getting to your goal (maintaining your desired physique), you need to fine-tune. I suggest adjusting your calorie needs up or down before changing your goal.

You need just as much leucine as a person whose goal is to get lean or build muscle. If you don't stimulate your muscle with leucine and use that muscle, you will lose it. Our sensitivity to leucine and its muscle-boosting effects decreases with age. The older we get, the more leucine we need to maintain muscle.

For our sample subject, let's consider a 45-year-old, 5-foot-6-inch woman who has reached a healthy weight of 140 pounds and wants to maintain it while living a relatively active lifestyle at an activity factor of 1.55.

BMR = 655 + (4.35 x weight in pounds)
+ (4.7 x height in inches) – (4.7 x age in years)

BMR= 655 + (4.35 x 140) + (4.7 x 66) – (4.7 x 45) = 655 + 609
+ 310.2 – 211.5 = 1363

1363 calories x activity factor of 1.55 = Total of 2112 calories per day

Thus, our 45-year-old woman needs 422 calories per meal, 28 LFPs, and a minimum of 28 grams of protein per meal (1 gram per pound of body weight divided by five meals: 140 ÷ 5 = 28).

Calories in 28 grams of protein = 112 calories
(28 x 4 calories per gram)

422 – 112 = 310 remaining calories. Health maintainers divide those remaining calories into 50% carbohydrates and 50% fats. Thus:

Carbs: 155 calories ÷ 4 calories per gram = 39 grams of carbs per meal

Fats: 155 calories ÷ 9 calories per gram= 17 grams of fat per meal

SAMPLE DIET AND EXERCISE PLAN FOR MAINTAINING HEALTH	
ACTIVITY	**DETAILS**
Breakfast	I cup 2% cottage cheese 2 slices of Ezekiel bread and I tablespoon olive oil–based butter substitute or natural peanut butter
Lunch	Grilled chicken breast sandwich with 3 ounces chicken breast, I ounce low-fat Swiss cheese, hamburger bun, avocado slices, and lettuce or spinach Piece of fruit
Dinner	4 ounces pork tenderloin 5 ounces yams Spinach and broccoli salad with olive oil

TYPICAL DAY:

The goal is 28 grams of protein, 39 grams of carbs, and 17 grams of fats adjusted for a leucine need of 28 LFPs.

Breakfast: A cup (8 ounces) of 2% cottage cheese provides 24 LFPs, 24 grams of protein, 4.8 grams of fat, and 10.4 grams of carbs. Two slices of Ezekiel bread supply 25 grams of carbs and 6.6 grams of additional protein. You can make up for the excess 24 calories (2 grams) of protein by cutting back on 2 grams of carbs or 1 gram of fat (when the excess is greater, remove the excess calories from carbs and fat equally). To get the rest of the fat (12.2 grams), you can either add 1 tablespoon of olive oil–based butter substitute or natural peanut butter. You could replace one slice of bread with frozen blueberries or pineapple added to the cottage cheese.

Lunch: The sandwich filling of 3 ounces of chicken breast and 1 ounce of low-fat Swiss cheese provides 30 LFPs, 33.3 grams of protein, and 4.1 grams of fat. A typical hamburger bun may have 20 grams of carbohydrate and 2 grams of fat. You can add avocado to reach your fat needs, and a piece of fruit will meet your remaining carb needs. Don't forget some lettuce or spinach—it's free.

Dinner: A 4-ounce serving of pork tenderloin provides nearly 28 LFPs, 33 grams of protein, and approximately 10 grams of fat. This leaves 7 grams of fat and the need for a carbohydrate source. A 5-ounce serving of yams will provide the needed carbohydrate of 39 grams, and some oil (1½ teaspoons) on a salad with spinach and broccoli will meet your fat needs.

Having a dessert now and then is okay. However, consider cutting back on some carbs and fats on those days, and don't go overboard with the dessert. You may also want some added time on the treadmill the next morning. If you can replace some of your fat and carbohydrate calories in your dinner, you can have a glass of wine. Wine is rich in polyphenols and, at one glass per day, has been proven to be beneficial to heart health.

The supplements you take as a health maintainer are completely dependent on your goals. If your goal is longevity, then added antioxidant supplements like curcumin/turmeric, resveratrol, quercetin, and ginger extracts can be beneficial.

EXERCISE TO MAINTAIN HEALTH

Anyone who is health conscious is probably already participating in regular physical activity. I hope that this activity consists of a combination of aerobic conditioning and resistance exercises with weights, machines, or your body weight. Aerobic conditioning improves cardiovascular health and breathing efficiency. Strength training helps maintain muscle as metabolic currency and skeletal support.

I recommend working out at least 3 or 4 days per week, although the ideal is 6 or 7 days per week. If your time is limited, perform your aerobic conditioning as part of your resistance training (for example, circuit training with little rest) or do some short high-intensity cardio before you lift. At a minimum, 2 days of lifting and 1 day of high-intensity interval training can help maintain muscle and cardiovascular function.

BUILD MUSCLE

Consider a 35-year-old, 5-foot-9-inch man who weighs 170 pounds and wants to put on 15 pounds of muscle. Let's calculate calorie and macronutrient needs based on the goal weight of 185 pounds. Our hypothetical man likes to train 5 days a week at a pretty high intensity, for an activity factor of 1.55. Thus, his total daily energy expenditure is:

BMR = 66 + (6.23 x goal weight in pounds) + (12.7 x height in Inches) – (6.8 x age in years)

$BMR = 66 + (6.23 \times 185) + (12.7 \times 69) - (6.8 \times 35) = 66 + 1152.55$
$+ 876.3 - 238 = 1856.85$

1856.85 calories x activity factor of 1.55 = 2878 calories per day

Since this man wants to gain muscle, add another 250 calories for a total of 3128 per day.

Thus, he needs 626 calories per meal, 37 LFPs, and a minimum of 37 grams of protein per meal.

Calories in 37 grams of protein = 148 calories
(37 x 4 calories per gram)

626 – 148 = 478 remaining calories. Muscle builders divide those remaining calories into 60% carbohydrates and 40% fats. Thus:

Carbs: 287 calories ÷ 4 calories per gram = 72 grams of carbs per meal

Fats: 191 calories ÷ 9 calories per gram = 21 grams of fats per meal

SAMPLE DIET AND EXERCISE PLAN FOR BUILDING MUSCLE		
TIME	**ACTIVITY**	**DETAILS**
7 a.m.	Breakfast	3 ounces egg yolks 8.7 ounces egg whites Oatmeal or 2 slices of Ezekiel bread
10 a.m.	Midmorning meal	Peanut or almond butter sandwich with Ezekiel bread Fruit shake with I banana or I cup blueberries and 2% milk
I p.m.	Lunch	6 ounces 85% fat ground beef I ounce yams I ounce brown rice Greens such as broccoli, kale, spinach, or asparagus
4 p.m.	60-minute workout	Weightlifting workout
5 p.m.	Post-workout nutrition	Shake with 40 grams whey protein, fruit, and coconut oil
7 p.m.	Dinner	4.4 ounces beef top sirloin steak Whole wheat pasta or rice with olive oil or cashews Greens such as broccoli, kale, spinach, or asparagus

> All weights of meat, fish, seafood, or poultry are cooked weights unless specified.

WEIGHT TRAINING AND AEROBICS

If your goal is to get lean, you can't be afraid of weights. Resistance training with weights, machines, or your body weight helps build and/or maintain muscle. It is especially important to stimulate muscle to grow when you're in a calorie-restricted state. By getting adequate amounts of leucine with each meal and especially post-workout, even a person whose goal is to get lean can build muscle.

Mobilizing fat to be burned can obviously be done with cardiovascular training on a bike, on the elliptical, on the track, or in the pool, but did you know that you can burn fat with weight training? Training with heavy weights is the classic example of an anaerobic exercise. "An" means "without" and "aerobic" means "air or oxygen." When you lift heavy weights with sufficient rest between sets, you usually don't get extraordinarily winded. You get a burn and fatigue in your muscle that brings you to exhaustion in relatively few reps. This process involves energy mechanisms in your muscle that don't require oxygen to burn fat as fuel.

Cardio is exercise that stimulates and improves the fitness of your heart. It is aerobic, meaning it requires oxygen to create fuel for muscle movement. Cardio can be done in many forms, but it usually involves low-resistance exercise using large muscle groups in repetitive movements. The ultimate objective of cardio is to improve cardiovascular health, efficiency, and performance while burning fat.

When you perform cardio, you elevate your heart rate and breathe more heavily with a corresponding elevation in energy expenditure. During this type of training, your body utilizes oxidative metabolism. That is, your body consumes oxygen in the process of burning fat stores to produce energy, and it produces and releases carbon dioxide (CO_2) from the lungs. This is why cardio is called aerobic exercise. It is a very energy-efficient process, and a well-trained person can do aerobic exercise for long periods.

Conversely, anaerobic exercise involves a higher intensity that uses stored carbohydrates for fuel and produces the painful lactic acid in your muscles that comes with the burn. Despite what many people think, the line between aerobic exercise and anaerobic exercise is blurred. Aerobic exercise can become anaerobic if the exercise becomes so intense that you are quickly exhausted and your lungs can't get enough oxygen to your muscle. For instance, if you run at a steady pace and then sprint to exhaustion, you have just converted aerobic exercise to anaerobic exercise. You know this has happened because you become short of breath and must rest from the pain in your muscle. If you aren't bringing in enough oxygen as you get short of breath, you can no longer acquire energy from oxidative metabolism. Anaerobic activity burns stored carbohydrates (glycogen) and energy stored as creatine phosphate.

You can blur this line and float between anaerobic and aerobic activity by keeping your workout moving between weight-training exercises. One way to do this is to create a circuit of three to five weight-training exercises that alternate from one muscle group to another. This way you can exhaust one muscle with relatively heavy weight (for example, failure at 10 to 12 reps) and then move to another muscle group and so on. Try making a circuit of squats, push-ups, and crunches. Going through this circuit five times with very little rest in between exercises will get your muscles pumped, your heart rate up, and your fat burning.

Consider mixing in some high-intensity intervals on the bike or treadmill with some weight-training exercises to boost your heart rate even higher. However, if you get to the point where you are struggling to speak because you are breathing too hard, you are probably not getting enough oxygen to your muscles to burn fat efficiently. Take a short break to let your heart rate come down, and then keep moving.

Visit YourGAINPlan.com for a Century Club Challenge designed to blur the lines between anaerobic weight training and aerobic conditioning.

TYPICAL DAY:

The goal is 37 grams of protein, 72 grams of carbs, and 21 grams of fats adjusted for a leucine need of 37 LFPs.

7 a.m. Breakfast. If you choose eggs* for breakfast, 1 ounce of egg whites has 2.9 LFPs, 3.1 grams of protein, and 0 grams of fat and carbs. An egg yolk has 3.9 LFPs per ounce, 4.5 grams of protein, 7.5 grams of fat, and 1 gram of carbs. Since your goal is 21 grams of fat, you can start with 3 ounces of egg yolks = 11.7 LFPs, 13.5 grams of protein, 22.5 grams of fat, and 3 grams of carbohydrate. This mildly overshoots the fat requirement but is within acceptable limits for someone who wants to gain muscle (but avoid overshooting by more than 5 grams of fat in a meal).

Now you need to use the remaining 25.3 LFPs, so 25.3 ÷ 2.9 LFPs in an egg white = 8.7 ounces of egg white. This gives you 27 grams of protein from egg white plus the 13.5 grams from the yolks for a total of 40.5 grams of protein (meeting your 37-gram protein requirement). Muscle builders can use extra protein calories without consequence. Add carbs to meet the 69 grams of carbs remaining. You can get them from a combination of fruit and oatmeal or two slices of Ezekiel bread.

Feel free to make an omelet and add greens as a free food; if you add cheese, take away the equivalent of an egg yolk from your fat or carbohydrate total.

10 a.m. Midmorning meal. This meal can be the same as breakfast, a similar lunch meal, or a protein bar or shake that meets your macronutrient needs.

As a muscle builder, you would shoot for 37 grams of whey protein for a total of 37 LFPs. You could add 1.5 ounces of peanuts (or almonds) for an additional 6.6 LFPs, 21 grams of fat, 11 grams of protein, and about 7 grams of carbs. Another option is to have a peanut butter or almond butter sandwich with Ezekiel bread for a total of 30 grams of carbs. This results in 9 extra grams of protein that can be accepted without consequence. A piece of fruit such as an unripe banana or a cup of blueberries in a shake can provide the needed carbs. Use 2% milk in the shake to replace some fruit carbs and nut butter fats if this is your preference.

1 p.m. Lunch. This meal can be the same as dinner or any of the other meals. I recommend meat or fish with a vegetable and a complex carb.

Let's say you choose beef flank steak, which has 6.3 LFPs per ounce with 7.9 grams of protein and 3.7 grams of fat. So, approximately 6 ounces of ground beef would give you 37.8 LFPs, 47.4 grams of protein, and 22.2 grams of fat. Now all you need to do is add some carbs. Yams have 7.8 grams per ounce, and brown rice 21.6 grams per ounce. A piece of fruit or even dairy like Greek yogurt or mozzarella cheese can replace some of the protein with fats and carbs needs.

Remember, incorporate some greens as they are a free food. Just don't use oil on them without removing the fats from the meat/fish or calories from the carb. (Account for fat-containing condiments when you make your protein choices.)

4 p.m. Afternoon workout. This is the time you go to the gym for a weightlifting workout. See the sample muscle-building exercise routine on page 132.

5 p.m. Post-workout nutrition. Consider a fast-absorbed protein such as whey protein isolates or hydrolysates. 40 grams of whey protein and a carb such as fruit or oatmeal added to your shake will help replenish glycogen stores and get insulin flowing to push nutrients into your muscle. If you plan to lift heavier weights or train for performance, then consider having half of your meal 30 minutes prior to training and the other half immediately afterward. Leave most of the fats for after your training. You can try medium chain triglyceride oils or coconut oil as a fat source in your shake.

7 p.m. Dinner. Here, you can repeat a similar meal to lunch or opt for a mix of proteins, fats, and carbs. Just 4.4 ounces of beef top sirloin steak provides 37 LFPs, 37 grams of protein, and 7 grams of fat. This leaves 72 grams of carbs and 14 grams of fat. You can have a bowl of whole wheat pasta with olive oil to meet your carbohydrate and fat needs. Adding olive or sunflower oil to a salad or choosing a fattier meat can help you meet your fat needs.

> If you are gaining weight too quickly or gaining more fat than you'd like, cut back on carbs by 10 grams per meal. The muscle-building diet plan is relatively carbohydrate rich, and as you get closer to your goals you will need to start moving toward a maintenance diet, which has a more equal ratio of fats and carbs without the 250 added calories per day.

If your goal is to build muscle, you really should consider including creatine monohydrate in your routine. If you have never taken a creatine supplement, try 10 to 20 grams per day (2.5 to 5 grams four times per day) for 5 days, and then stay at 5 grams per day afterward. Also, include a whey protein isolate shake after training. Although a whole food meal is okay for every meal, whey protein—with its rapid digestion and absorption of highly concentrated leucine—will turn on muscle growth quickly after your intense training. Additionally, get some of your fats from fish oil, which has been shown to assist in turning on muscle protein synthesis.

MUSCLE-BUILDING EXERCISE ROUTINE

Here is my favorite muscle-building 5-day training split. A repetition range of 6 to 12 reps per set helps to build strength and muscle. Pick four or five exercises per body part and perform 4 or 5 sets per exercise. Pyramid your weights with each exercise (start light in first set, go heavier in a couple more sets, then finish with a lighter weight). Let the first couple of sets build up your comfort with the movement at 10 to 12 reps, and follow with 2 hard "working sets" burning out at 6 to 8 reps. Working sets are the ones that really help to build muscle and strength. A final set of 10 reps can be done with a slightly lighter weight to exhaustion or even with a drop set or assisted reps.

DAY	EXERCISE
Day 1: Chest	Incline bench, machine press, pec flies, dips
Day 2: Back	Chin-ups, seated rows, deadlifts, wide-grip pull-downs, back extensions
Day 3: Legs	Squats, leg presses, walking lunges, leg extensions, leg curls, calf raises
Day 4: Relative rest	Stretching, low-intensity cardio
Day 5: Shoulders, abs	Military presses, rear deltoid flies, lateral raises, leg raises, crunches
Day 6: Biceps, triceps	Barbell curls, concentration curls, hammer curls, push-downs, kickbacks
Day 7: Relative rest	Stretching, low-intensity cardio

GET LEAN

The sample diet and exercise plan that follows is for our hypothetical woman who is 35 years old, stands 5 feet 4 inches tall, has 20% body fat, and weighs 130 pounds but wants to be 120 pounds and leaner.

SAMPLE DIET AND EXERCISE PLAN
FOR GETTING LEAN

TIME	ACTIVITY	DETAILS
6 a.m.	30-minute fasted morning cardio	3 to 5 days a week
7 a.m.	Breakfast	2 ounces egg yolks 5.6 ounces egg whites I slice of Ezekiel bread or I ounce dry weight oatmeal
10 a.m.	Midmorning meal	Same as breakfast or similar lunch meal or protein bar/shake
I p.m.	Lunch	4 ounces farmed salmon 2.5 ounces yams Greens such as broccoli, kale, spinach, or asparagus
4 p.m.	60-minute workout	Weightlifting or circuit training or HIIT exercise
5 p.m.	Post-workout nutrition	20 grams whey protein I ounce peanuts 3 ounces unripe (yellow not black) banana
7 p.m.	Dinner	3 ounces beef top sirloin steak 3 ounces brown rice I ounce low-fat Swiss cheese Greens such as broccoli, kale, spinach, or asparagus

TYPICAL DAY:

The goal for each meal is 24 grams of protein, 15 grams of fats, and 22 grams of carbs adjusted for a leucine need of 24 LFPs.

6 a.m. Fasted cardio. Get up for your 30 minutes of fasted morning cardio (3 to 5 days per week). Your goal is to reach a heart rate of about 140 beats per minute for half of your session. Do not eat before you exercise. However, water, black coffee, or HMB and/or a fat-burning supplement prior to your cardio is allowed.

7 a.m. Breakfast. If you choose eggs* for breakfast, here's the breakdown of nutrients and LFPs:

FOOD (I OUNCE)	LFPs	PROTEIN	FAT	CARBS
Egg white	2.9	3.1 g	0 g	0 g
Egg yolk	3.9	4.5 g	7.5 g	I g

Since your goal is only 15 grams of fat per meal, you can start with 2 ounces of egg yolks = 7.8 LFPs, 9 grams of protein, 15 grams of fat, and 2 grams of carbs. Since you still need 16.2 LFPs to get to your goal of 24 LFPs, add 5.6 ounces of fat-free egg whites. To determine the amount of egg whites, divide 16.2 LFPs by the number of LFPs in 1 ounce of egg whites.

16.2 ÷ 2.9 LFPs in 1 ounce egg white = 5.6 ounces egg whites

This gives you 17.4 grams of protein from 5.6 ounces of egg whites plus 9 grams from 2 ounces of egg yolks for a total of 26.4 grams of protein (meeting your 24-gram protein requirement).

Since you are 2.4 grams of protein over the protein requirement, remove those grams from carbohydrates, leaving you with 17.6 grams of carbs for the meal. You can get this from a slice of Ezekiel bread or an ounce of oatmeal.

Feel free to make an omelet and add greens as a free food; if you add cheese, take away the equivalent of an egg yolk from your fat or carbohydrate total.

10 a.m. Midmorning meal. This meal can be the same as breakfast, a similar lunch meal, or a protein bar or shake that meets your macronutrient needs.

Shoot for 20 grams of whey protein for a total of 20 LFPs. You could add an ounce of peanuts or almonds for an additional 4 LFPs, 14 grams of fat, approximately 6 grams of protein, and about 5 grams of carbs. This results in 2 extra grams of protein removed from carbs for 20 grams of carbs minus the 5 grams from the nuts = 15 grams of carbs remaining.

This is a time where, for the sake of simplification, I would shift the unconsumed 15 grams of carbs to either lunch or the post-workout meal, have a small piece of fruit (such as 3 ounces of unripe banana in a shake), or just chalk it up as a slight caloric deficit for getting lean.

1 p.m. Lunch. This meal can be the same as dinner or any of the other meals. I recommend meat or fish with a vegetable and a complex carb.

Let's say you choose salmon. Farmed salmon has 5.1 LFPs per ounce with 6.3 grams of protein and 3.5 grams of fat. So, 4.7 ounces of farmed salmon would give you 24 LFPs, 29.6 grams of protein, and 16.5 grams of fat. If you subtract the additional protein from the carbohydrates, this leaves 16.4 grams of carbs, and 1.5 grams of extra fat. 2.0 ounces of yams will give you another 15.6 grams of carbs and 1 gram of protein for a pretty complete meal that meets your macronutrient needs with a very little bit of extra fat. Remember, incorporate some greens as they are a free food. Just don't use oil on them without removing the fats from the meat/fish or calories from the carbs. In other words, if you like oil on your vegetables, you'll need to pick a leaner protein like wild salmon.

> Foods like salmon will have variable amounts of fats in every serving of even the same fish. More might have cooked off or you might just get a little marbling. These diets don't have to be an exact science, you just need to be as close as possible. If you get your macronutrients within 3 to 5 grams of your goal then you are doing well. Shoot for optimizing the leucine content. If you are trying to get lean, slightly undershoot fat and carbs if possible; if trying to build muscle, err toward overshooting.

4 p.m. Afternoon workout. This is the time you go to the gym for up to 60 minutes of weightlifting, circuit training, or HIIT exercise (3 to 5 days per week). Consider trying a circuit like my Century

Club Challenge found at YourGAINPlan.com. You could also take a traditional bodybuilding approach to weightlifting or mix up some weights, HIIT, machines, and plyometrics.

5 p.m. Post-workout nutrition. Consider a fast-absorbed protein such as whey protein isolates or hydrolysates. 20 grams of whey protein with 1 ounce of peanuts and 3 ounces of unripe banana will give you 24 LFPs, 26 grams of protein, 14 grams of fats, and approximately 20 grams of carbs, closely meeting your goals.

Having a little more post-workout carbs is okay as the body tends to utilize those carbs more to restore muscle glycogen than to create fat. Avoid eating any carbs before your training to keep the fat-burning machinery running. If you plan to lift heavier weights or train for performance, then consider having half of your meal 30 minutes prior to training and the other half immediately afterward.

7 p.m. Dinner. You can opt for a similar meal to lunch or a different mix of proteins, fats, and carbs. Consider reducing your carbs in this meal and adding the calories to fat or protein if you would like to avoid sugar storage to burn more fat with morning cardio.

If you pick a meat like beef top sirloin steak (fat-trimmed lean cut) you can get by with 3 ounces for 25.5 LFPs, 25 grams of protein, and 4.5 grams of fat. This leaves 21 grams of carbs and 10.5 grams of fats. You can have 3 ounces of brown rice for 21.6 grams of carbs, and maybe add a little (1 ounce) of low-fat Swiss cheese to your green leafy salad or meat for 8.4 LFPs, 7.2 grams of protein, 1.4 grams of fats, and 1.2 grams of carbs. Now you have exceeded your LFPs and protein, but not fat or carbs. If you would like to be closer to your fat intake goal, consider a fattier meat such as ground beef, ground turkey, or fish.

For those in the "get lean" category, accept a little more calorie deficit at first. If you find you are losing too much weight or are too hungry, you can be stricter in meeting your macronutrient goals.

FASTED CARDIO

One of the controversies in nutrition and exercise is whether or not to consume carbohydrates prior to fat-burning exercise. Clearly, a person should consume carbs before exercise meant to improve performance or in competition, but the situation is different when the goal is to burn fat. Anyone trying to lose fat usually cuts calories from carbs and/or fats. These reductions can put a strain on hard-earned muscle and risk unwanted loss of muscle.

A substantial portion of energy production during endurance comes from burning fat. When your diet is higher in protein and fat with lower carbs, your muscle more effectively utilizes fat to spare muscle glycogen (glucose stores). Furthermore, endurance training improves the muscle's ability to use fat for energy, sparing muscle glycogen and protein. If your diet is high in carbohydrates, the percentage of carbs used during endurance exercise increases. Burning glucose for energy increases progressively with exercise intensity, whereas the most efficient fat burning happens during exercise at 70% of maximum heart rate (HR_{max}), which is measured in beats per minute (bpm).

Maximum heart rate = 220 – your age

For our hypothetical 35-year-old woman: (220 – 35) x 70% = 130 b pm

This measurement technique is often underestimated for healthier individuals, so I recommend a HR_{max} of 135 to 140 bpm if you train regularly (increase your goal by 5 to 10 bpm).

Fat is readily available for energy after a night of sleep, as liver glycogen stores are depleted by the overnight fast. Thus, there is less glucose available to burn as fuel and the body must tap other sources of fuel like fat. During cardiovascular exercise, the body releases fat from stores—resulting in more fat available for working muscles. If you consume a carb-rich meal before exercise, glucose becomes the preferred fuel and fat release enzymes are shut down by the rise in insulin. Insulin commands that glucose in the blood be converted into stores of fat and glycogen. What all of this means is that if you're exercising to burn fat, then consuming glucose (carbs or sugar) before exercising is counterproductive to your goal. Research supports that you'll burn more fat when you're in a fasted state than after you've eaten.

Traditionally, the teaching is that if your endurance training is meant to make you stronger, faster, or more conditioned for distance rather than for burning fat, then you should spare your muscle and fat by consuming carbs, at a minimum after training. However, fasting before endurance training can provide a stimulus for improvements in fat burning, and may even be considered as an adjunctive training technique in those at the top of their game. That is, fasted endurance training improves the contribution of fats used in energy production during endurance training.

Fasted training improves your muscle's efficiency to burn fat more than the same exercise done with a high-carb intake. Perhaps more important for the low-carb dieter, fasted endurance training prevents the drop in blood glucose seen in exercise after a carbohydrate meal. This avoids the crash that can occur when training after consuming sugars or carbs.

Although some studies show that fasted cardio can lead to greater muscle breakdown for energy, the data is not as applicable to the Leucine Factor dieter. Most studies that have examined the effects of fasting did not incorporate increased protein intake, anabolic weight training, and anabolic nutritional supplementation. Weight-training exercise encourages muscle growth, and supplements like creatine monohydrate and HMB have anti-catabolic effects on muscle. Taking an HMB supplement prior to your fasted cardio in the morning can help spare muscle breakdown during cardio.

If you want the fat-burning machinery to keep working longer, a low-carb (less than 100 grams per day) or very low-carb (less than

50 grams per day) diet will maximize mobilization of fat. Based on this science, I recommend combining fasted cardio at moderate intensities before breakfast with a low-carb diet when your goal is to lose body fat quickly. When starches are a part of your diet, you must time their consumption to spare muscle and lose fat. For instance, I recommend consuming starchy carbs after your weight-training session. The key is to avoid situations in which consumed carbs are most likely to be stored as fat. That means no carbs before periods of relative inactivity such as rest or sleep.

8

RECIPES FOR THE LEUCINE FACTOR DIET

These are my favorite recipes as made by Chef Donato Coluccio. They incorporate great sources of leucine that taste great. Now that you have learned how to eat to live and attain your goals, you can live to eat these healthy foods. Choose your quantities as they fit your macronutrient needs.

PORK TENDERLOIN

	Amount	LFPs	Protein per ounce	Fats per ounce
Pork Tenderloin	I ounce	6.8	8.3 g	2.4 g

INGREDIENTS

1 tablespoon extra virgin olive oil

½ tablespoon fresh lime juice

½ tablespoon fresh lemon juice

1 tablespoon cider vinegar

1 green onion, minced

1 clove garlic, minced

1 tablespoon ground coriander

1 tablespoon thyme leaf

1 tablespoon cilantro, minced

black pepper to taste

1 pork tenderloin, trimmed of visible fat

salt to taste

INSTRUCTIONS

Place all the ingredients except the pork and the salt in a baking pan, and mix well. Put in the pork, and marinate for a minimum of 1 hour and a maximum of 4 hours, turning the meat every half hour or so. At grill time, drain the pork but save the marinade for basting. Salt the pork before grilling. Grill to medium, about 3 minutes on each side. Remove from the grill, and let rest for 10 minutes before slicing. Serve with yams and a leafy green vegetable such as spinach or kale.

Note: Start with a high flame on one side of the grill to sear, and a lower flame on the other side to finish, depending on wind and weather. The larger the meat, the longer you should marinate it. The tougher the cut, the longer and slower it should cook.

SAVORY BROCCOLI

Broccoli on its own is a free food on the Leucine Factor Diet. Create a scrumptious meal or side dish by combining the broccoli with egg and Parmesan cheese, rich sources of leucine. Use reduced-fat cheese or egg whites to minimize the calories. Note: One extra-large whole egg is about 2 ounces.

	Amount	LFPs	Protein per ounce	Fat per ounce
Reduced-fat Parmesan Cheese	I ounce	8.5	5.7 g	5.7 g
Egg	I ounce	3.3	3.5 g	2.7 g

INGREDIENTS

1 bunch broccoli crowns

6 eggs

2 cups grated reduced-fat Parmesan cheese, divided

1 tablespoon garlic powder

4 tablespoons chopped parsley

olive oil for sautéing

lemon for squeezing

salt and pepper to taste

INSTRUCTIONS

Blanch the broccoli crowns in boiling water, and then shock them in ice water. Beat the eggs, 1 cup of the cheese, the garlic, and the parsley until the mixture is fluffy. Heat olive oil in a pan over moderate heat. Dip the broccoli in the egg mixture, and sauté until golden brown. Drain on paper towels, and serve with a squeeze of lemon on top and the remaining cup of Parmesan cheese on the side. Season with salt and pepper to taste.

FRENCH TOAST

French toast doesn't have to be bad for you. Using whole grain sprouted bread like Ezekiel bread is a healthier way to enjoy this breakfast treat. Cut back on the yolks or cream to reduce the amount of fat. Accompany the meal with a whey protein smoothie to get more protein and concentrated leucine. This recipe makes a large yield; save leftovers in the fridge and pop leftover slices in the toaster for a quick breakfast the next day. Note: One whole egg is about 2 ounces.

	Amount	LFPs	Protein per ounce	Fat per ounce
Egg	I ounce	3.3	3.5 g	2.7 g
2% milk	I ounce	I	I.I g	0.6 g

INGREDIENTS

8 eggs

1 tablespoon cinnamon

1 tablespoon nutmeg

2 tablespoons vanilla extract

½ cup 2% milk (use half-and-half for more fat)

8 slices thick multigrain Ezekiel bread

dry steel-cut oatmeal for coating

coconut oil for sautéing

INSTRUCTIONS

Beat the eggs, cinnamon, nutmeg, vanilla, and milk well. Dip each slice of bread in the egg mixture for a minute, and then coat with the oats. Heat the coconut oil in a pan over medium heat. Sauté the French toast until crispy brown. Serve with toppings of your choice, such as berries or toasted almonds.

OPEN-FACED TUNA MELT

Fresh tuna steak is a great way to get more leucine and protein in your diet. Add the low-fat cheese of your choice, such as reduced-fat Parmesan, and you have a meal that delivers plenty of leucine for your needs.

	Amount	LFPs	Protein per ounce	Fat per ounce
Tuna (yellowfin) steak	I ounce	6.4	8.3 g	0.2 g
Reduced-fat Parmesan cheese	I ounce	8.5	5.7 g	5.7 g

INGREDIENTS

4 (4-ounce) fresh tuna steak fillets

1 tablespoon minced tarragon

1 teaspoon chopped cilantro

4 tablespoons grated reduced-fat Parmesan cheese

2 tablespoons Dijon mustard

1 tablespoon lemon zest

1 tablespoon lemon juice

pepper to taste

INSTRUCTIONS

Let the tuna sit at room temperature for 10 minutes. Mix the tarragon and cilantro with the cheese, Dijon mustard, lemon zest, lemon juice, and pepper. Rub the tuna with the herb mix, and grill over moderate heat until medium rare, about 2 minutes on each side. The herbs and cheese should brown but not burn. Serve on Ezekiel bread, an English muffin, or a bed of roasted cauliflower with spinach or arugula and tomatoes.

GROUND TURKEY AND SPINACH FRITTATA

Combining eggs, cheese, and ground turkey is a delicious way to meet your leucine and protein needs. A frittata is also a good choice for premade breakfasts for an on-the-go lifestyle. Note: One whole egg is about 2 ounces.

	Amount	LFPs	Protein per ounce	Fat per ounce
Egg	I ounce	3.3	3.5 g	2.7 g
Ground turkey, 93% fat	I ounce	4.4	5.3 g	2.4 g
Ground turkey breast, 97% fat	I ounce	5.3	8.5 g	0.6 g
Reduced-fat Parmesan cheese	I ounce	8.5	5.7 g	5.7 g

INGREDIENTS

8 ounces 93% fat ground turkey or 97% fat ground turkey breast

½ cup diced sweet onion

1½ cups chopped and blanched spinach, asparagus, or other green vegetable

8 eggs, lightly beaten

¼ cup grated reduced-fat Parmesan cheese

¼ cup basket cheese

salt and pepper to taste

INSTRUCTIONS

Preheat the oven to 350°F. Coat an ovenproof nonstick pan with cooking spray. Over medium-high heat, sauté the turkey, onion, and vegetable until cooked. Add the eggs and cheese, and sauté on low to make sure the mixture doesn't stick. Place the pan in the oven to finish the frittata. Remove when cooked through and light brown, approximately 5 minutes. Season with salt and pepper to taste. Serve immediately or refrigerate for later use.

ESPRESSO RUB SIRLOIN

Steak is a great way to get a high-protein meal with plenty of leucine. Lean beef and bison steaks are very concentrated sources of leucine. Boost your metabolism a little by adding some espresso beans. This recipe from Chef Donato Coluccio is one of my favorites. With some Parmesan cheese, this meal is guaranteed to meet your leucine goals.

	Amount	LFPs	Protein per ounce	Fat per ounce
Beef top sirloin	1 ounce	8.5	8.3 g	1.5 g
Reduced-fat Parmesan cheese	1 ounce	8.5	5.7 g	5.7 g

INGREDIENTS

4 (12-ounce) beef top sirloin steaks

¼ cup ground espresso beans

2 tablespoons cocoa powder

1 tablespoon dry mustard

¼ teaspoon red pepper flakes

2 tablespoons coarse ground black pepper

¼ cup garlic powder

1 tablespoon onion powder

1 teaspoon ground cloves

smoked kosher salt to taste

1 tablespoon raw sugar or ½ Splenda

¼ cup grated reduced-fat Parmesan cheese

2 cups creamed pearl onion

INSTRUCTIONS

Rub the steaks all over with the ground espresso, seasonings, spices, and cheese. Cook the steaks on a medium high–flamed outdoor or indoor grill to the desired doneness, then serve with the creamed onions. I prefer medium rare (warm red center). There should be about ½ cup of the onions per steak, or add to the recipe if you want more.

9

NOT JUST ANOTHER DIET PROGRAM

The common thread among all weight loss programs is that they are based on calorie reduction, on the principle that dieters consume fewer calories than they expend. However, the majority of programs fail because they are temporary or unsustainable. When people talk about "dieting," the implication is that a diet is something you start and then eventually stop. Most of us have been tricked into believing that we can go on a diet, get fit, and then go off the diet and stay fit. Even though there are more diet programs in the United States than ever before, the rates of obesity and associated diseases continue to rise.

To overcome this mindset about dieting, we need to understand that diet is an inherent part of life and must be maintained just like teeth, cleanliness, and mental well-being. Societal pressures make this a very difficult proposition. Everywhere you turn are advertisements for or easy access to fast foods and processed treats.

One of the biggest mistakes people make when embarking on one of these diet programs is that they do too much too quickly and try to starve the fat off. They might see rapid results at first, but they soon relapse. The problem does not arise from a lack of personal desire, but from a deeply rooted evolutionary survival mechanism against starvation that zaps strength and willpower.

Research published in the *New England Journal of Medicine* supports that changes in hormone levels make it very difficult to stay on diets with significant calorie restrictions. Even after a brief 10-week diet, our bodies produce hormones that increase hunger for up to a year later! Furthermore, mental and physical stresses lead to changes in the brain that make fatty and sugary foods more appealing. Starving ourselves is truly counterproductive.

Starvation dieting also results in a loss of valuable muscle mass— what I call metabolic currency. Muscles are little furnaces that burn fat and sugar to create movement and warmth. Being active with more muscle helps us to stay metabolically healthy. When we starve muscle, we lose muscle. Once we lose muscle, it is much easier for our bodies to store more fat, because fewer calories can be burned. Starvation dieting leads to a "skinny fat" body; that is, someone who may be normal weight but weak and flabby.

The fact is that you have to permanently change the way you eat and combine that shift with comprehensive lifestyle changes, including stress management and muscle-building exercise. Return to old habits and the weight will pile on again, perhaps even faster than before.

GOT GOALS?

A dream becomes a goal when you give it a deadline. – Anonymous

One of the keys to making healthy lifestyle changes like those presented in this book is to determine your goals and anything hindering you from attaining them. Your goals will essentially bring about changes in your life.

Making deliberate changes creates wisdom. Change presents a chance to learn something new. The mistakes that occur along the way are inevitable, but you will learn from mistakes and grow from them. Mistakes and recovery from them can lead to a closer relationship with loved ones and new friends as they reach out to help you. Challenges will arise, and you overcome them as long as you have the right tools. If you embark on a journey toward a new goal without a map, your chances of success diminish.

I recommend reading the book *Who Moved My Cheese?* by Spencer Johnson. You will learn about the mice Hem and Haw, who are stuck in a rut because they became complacent with mediocrity and dependence. Once you realize that you need to change you need to build a plan and you are doing that now by reading *The Leucine Factor Diet.*

I'm always amazed by how many people have never sat down for 30 minutes and put their goals on paper. It could be as simple as jotting down things that you are going to do that day, or as complex as lifelong dreams and aspirations. Most people have spent more time making grocery lists than they have examining their goals for personal growth.

Where are you starting from? Where are you going? What are some of your goals? Write one of them down and turn your ethereal thoughts into written word. Start with just one goal until you get a grasp of the process. Be very specific in detailing your goal.

End goal: _____

(Example: 150 pounds)

Starting point: _____

(Example: 190 pounds)

Smallest manageable component of your goal:

_____

(Example: 1 pound per week)

Today's goals: _____

(Example: Eat 250 fewer calories)

Time required each day: _____

(Example: 1 hour at the gym, 30 minutes of meal prep)

This week's goals: _____

(Example: Lose 1 pound)

This month's goals: _____

(Example: Lose 4 pounds)

This year's goals: _____

(Example: Reach 150 pounds)

Lifelong goals: _____

_____

_____

(Example: Make sustainable changes to maintain my new weight)

When you set a goal, basically you are putting together an action plan. Once you have determined that your destination will be rewarding, your goal is the main motivator for keeping you on the road to success, and small accomplishments along the way will refuel your motivation tank. If you don't truly believe that attaining your goal will be rewarding, you may be quick to turn around and go home. You need to be honest with yourself. Write down the pros and cons of reaching your goal, and make sure that the destination is something you really desire. If your heart isn't into it, you will fail.

Pros of attaining your goal: _____

_____

_____

_____

_____

(Example: Less joint pain, more energy, wearing my skinny jeans)

Cons of attaining your goal: _____

_____

_____

_____

_____

(Example: Less going out to bars, less eating out, more time at the gym)

Just as you need to plan for rest from difficult training in the gym (such as 5 days on and 1 day off), you need to plan for rest and setbacks in attaining your goal. You need to step back and try to predict the obstacles you might encounter along the way. List some obstacles and how you might overcome them:

Obstacles: **Solutions:**

1. _____   _____

_____   _____

_____   _____

2. _____   _____

_____   _____

_____   _____

3. _____   _____

_____   _____

_____   _____

WHY PROCRASTINATE?

Distress about the work ahead or fear of failure can lead to procrastination. Procrastination is effectively putting off the inevitable in order to be more comfortable in the present. Unfortunately, as a deadline approaches, procrastination compounds the stress associated with getting the job done. Often, procrastination leads to subpar work and missed deadlines.

Many people feel immobilized by the stress of a deadline. They feel that they need to wait until they are in the mood to be productive. It is a common misconception that motivation or desire to work precedes productivity. Successful people know, and I have learned, that making yourself busy leads to motivation to do more work. If you wait until you feel like doing work, chances are you will never start the work. Taking action in work, especially in stressful and demanding tasks, is always difficult to do; otherwise it would be called play. However, the more you do, the more you will feel like doing, as you see the light at the end of the tunnel. Action begets action...it's the physics of the universe. Once you get an object moving, it will stay in motion until it is impeded by an outside force. At that point, it will pivot to a new course.

Newton's first law of motion: An object at rest stays at rest and an object in motion stays in motion unless acted upon by an external force. Your dreams and desires are the external force that move you from rest to motion.

It is important to recognize the stressors associated with achieving a goal. Work will be involved, and the process won't always be smooth and straightforward; your motion will be acted on by outside forces. However, rising to challenges and overcoming obstacles lead to personal growth, creativity, and intimacy. The sooner you accept that you'll encounter frustrations, the sooner you will be able to set off on a new course and complete your task. If you have a low tolerance for frustration and need to do everything perfectly, you will be paralyzed by your own expectations of yourself.

Nobody else in the world believes that you will always be perfect, so why would you? —Anonymous

Perfectionism can be a precursor of procrastination, and the more you procrastinate, the more difficult it becomes to make the project perfect. I have suffered from this form of procrastination. It is fine to have high standards in a healthy pursuit of excellence; I certainly do. However, if you base your self-esteem on the idea that everything you do must be perfect, you will lack motivation. Plan to be more motivated by the creative process and the small successes that come with overcoming challenges.

STEPS TO OVERCOME PROCRASTINATION

If you are procrastinating, whether the task is to finish a project, go to the gym, lose weight, or prepare for a contest, you need to analyze your situation objectively. Here are four steps to overcome procrastination.

1. WRITE DOWN THE PROS AND CONS OF PROCRASTINATING

The advantages of procrastinating are obvious: You can play more, eat more sweets, go out with friends, and so on. However, the cons will take a little more thought and likely will be eye-opening. In this process, you must be honest with yourself about whether you really have the desire to complete the task.

2. BUILD A DOABLE ACTION PLAN

Make a timeline to start your goal, not to finish it. If your goal has a deadline, be realistic in writing down how long you think it will take to accomplish. For example, you may realize that it will take 30 minutes of your day each day, 5 days a week for 4 weeks. Devoting 30 minutes a day may be easier than trying to find 10 hours in a single day to work on your goal. If you make the block of time too large, it can sap your motivation. It seems more painful to have to work for 2 hours rather than a smaller, 30-minute block.

Remember, 1 hour is only 4.2% of the day.

3. USE PMA: POSITIVE MENTAL ATTITUDE

Identify the negative thoughts that go through your head when you think about completing your goal. Are they reasonable? Would one of your friends think the same way? By writing down your thoughts, hopefully you will see the self-deception that is leading you to procrastinate. Being positive and realistic will push you forward in carrying out your action plan.

4. REWARD YOURSELF

You need to accept accomplishments, no matter how small, as successes. Even overcoming an obstacle such as recovering from a setback deserves self-recognition for the valuable lesson learned.

CONCLUSION

Now, take a deep breath! You have just gotten through a book that is a culmination of years of research and personal experience with dieting and nutrition. As a reminder, here are the main points of the Leucine Factor Diet.

1. Goal-oriented dieting must be a lifestyle. Make healthy nutrition a habit. Prepare your meals in advance to follow the five-meals-a-day plan (5-MAD).

2. There are essential fats and essential amino acids that we can't live without.

3. Eat all the green vegetables you want!

4. Shop the periphery of the grocery store. Spend equal amounts of time in the produce, meat, fish, poultry, egg, and dairy sections. Avoid overprocessed and aggressively promoted foods.

5. Look for hidden kryptonite in your foods. Sugar makes us weak. It comes in many forms; see Check Your Ingredients List on page 160.

6. If you eat sugar, make sure it is packaged the way nature intended, with lots of fiber—in the form of whole fruits, but eat them in moderation.

7. All proteins aren't created equal. Optimize the leucine content of your meals.

8. Take a daily multivitamin with minerals as a nutritional safety blanket.

9. To augment your foods, choose nutritional supplements based on your goals. Whey protein, creatine, fish oil, vitamin D$_3$, and HMB all improve muscle mass, function, and metabolism.

10. Practice everything in moderation, including moderation. Enjoy your new lifestyle, but allow for some fun now and then.

Use this book as a reference. You will likely need to go back and review some sections. If you remembered everything in this book, I would be in awe. The leucine, calorie, and macronutrient calculations may seem impossible now, but with some practice and use of the Leucine Factor Diet phone app, the diet should become a habit instead of work.

Remember, this diet is supposed to be in flux just as your life is, with its ups and downs. There aren't any calculations or estimates of energy expenditure or calorie needs that won't have some degree of numerical error for each individual. By grading your progress either by feelings of energy or fatigue, the scale, the mirror, your body fat percentage, or any other health metric, you will know if you need to adjust your calories up or down.

If you are losing weight too quickly or not gaining weight fast enough, add some calories to your plan. If you want to lose weight a little more quickly or find yourself gaining when you want to lose, cut your calories back a bit. Make very small adjustments unless you are seeing drastic problems. On that note, if you are seeing dramatic problems with this diet, please consult a health care professional.

A diet plan without exercise will not succeed. Activity deficiency is just as detrimental to your health as smoking. We all need to keep moving. Find time to exercise in the mornings before the rest of your household wakes up. Locate a gym that is on your way home from work. Set goals and look for gym or work buddies to help hold you accountable to your exercise plan.

Knowing that you have to keep moving, remember that resistance exercise builds muscle. The Leucine Factor Diet is meant to help you maintain or build muscle for metabolic currency, mobility, and longevity. Adding resistance exercise that stimulates muscle and works hand in hand with leucine will keep you on track. These exercises include lifting weights, calisthenics, CrossFit, gymnastics, Pilates, and the list goes on. Work against gravity and you will build muscle and bone density to keep your body moving.

Be prepared for distractions from your plan. By familiarizing yourself with leucine-rich foods and healthy food combinations on the Leucine Factor Diet phone app and the list on page 161, you will be able to make your leucine-rich meals in advance and have them ready for life's unscheduled events. Invest in food storage containers and make your meals every Sunday. Keep a list of meals handy for when you eat out. Remember, most restaurants can cook what you want. You just have to know what to ask for—for example, Give me a chicken breast with steamed broccoli and an arugula salad with an oil and vinegar dressing; I'd like a cheeseburger, no bun, and a baked potato without butter; I'd like a house salad with salmon on top. Don't be afraid to ask for what you know your body wants.

Good luck in your pursuit of lifelong health and longevity. Visit LeucineFactor.com for updates to the diet, recipes, and conversations with me. Live well, and be #BetterThanYesterdaysSelf.

CHECK YOUR INGREDIENTS LIST

HIDDEN SUGARS

- agave nectar
- Barbados sugar
- barley malt
- beet sugar
- brown sugar
- buttered syrup
- cane juice crystals
- cane sugar
- caramel
- confectioner's sugar
- corn syrup and corn syrup solids
- carob syrup
- castor sugar
- date sugar
- dehydrated cane juice
- demerara sugar
- dextran
- dextrose
- diatase
- diastatic malt
- ethyl maltol
- evaporated cane juice
- fructose
- fruit juice
- fruit juice concentrate
- galactose
- glucose
- glucose solids
- golden sugar
- golden syrup
- grape sugar
- high fructose corn syrup
- honey
- icing sugar
- invert sugar
- lactose
- maltodextrin
- maltose
- malt syrup
- maple syrup
- molasses
- muscovado sugar
- panocha
- raw sugar
- refiner's syrup
- rice syrup
- sorbitol
- sorghum syrup
- sucrose
- treacle

ARTIFICIAL SWEETENERS

- acesulfame K
- aspartame (Nutrasweet)
- neotame
- saccharin
- sucralose (Splenda)

SUGAR ALCOHOLS/ POLYOLS

- D-tagatose
- erythritol
- glycerol
- hydrogenated starch
- hydrolysates
- isomalt (Palatinit)
- lactitol
- maltitol
- mannitol
- polydextrose
- sorbitol
- xylitol

APPENDIX

LEUCINE FACTOR PREFERRED FOODS						
FOOD (I-OUNCE SERVING)	LEUCINE (GRAMS)	PROTEIN (GRAMS)	FAT (GRAMS)	CARBS (GRAMS)	CALORIES	LFPs
MEAT						
Beef Fillet (lean)	0.89	8.7	1.3	0	46.5	8.9
Beef Flank Steak	0.63	7.9	3.7	0	64.9	6.3
Beef Top Round Steak (fat trimmed)	0.9	8.5	I	0	43	9.I
Beef Top Sirloin Steak	0.85	8.3	1.5	0	46.7	8.5
Beef (ground, 85%)	0.6I	7.9	4.3	0	70.3	6.I
Beef (ground, 95%)	0.64	8.3	2.I	0	52.I	6.4
Bison Top Round	0.73	8.6	1.4	0	47	7.3
Bison Top Sirloin Steak	0.68	8	I.6	0	46.4	6.8
Lamb Chop (neck)	0.69	8.9	4.4	0	75.2	6.9
Lamb Lean Shoulder	0.78	I0.I	4	0	76.4	7.8
Ostrich (top loin)	0.65	7.9	I.I	0	4I.5	6.5

LEUCINE FACTOR PREFERRED FOODS

FOOD (1-OUNCE SERVING)	LEUCINE (GRAMS)	PROTEIN (GRAMS)	FAT (GRAMS)	CARBS (GRAMS)	CALORIES	LFPs
Pork Tenderloin (chops, lean)	0.68	8.3	2.4	0	54.8	6.8
Veal (lean boneless breast)	0.68	8.6	2.8	0	59.6	6.8
Veal (loin)	0.68	8.6	4.9	0	78.5	6.8
SEAFOOD						
Cod (Atlantic)	0.53	6.5	0.2	0	27.8	5.3
Crab (cooked)	0.53	6.7	0.4	0	30.4	5.3
Lobster	0.39	5.4	0.2	0	23.4	3.9
Mahi Mahi	0.55	6.7	0.3	0	29.5	5.5
Orange Roughy	0.51	6.4	0.25	0	27.85	5.1
Salmon (Atlantic, wild)	0.58	7.2	2.1	0	47.7	5.8
Salmon (farmed)	0.51	6.3	3.5	0	56.7	5.1
Scallops	0.35	5.8	0.2	1.5	31	3.5
Sea Bass	0.54	6.7	0.7	0	33.1	5.4
Shrimp	0.55	6.5	0.5	0.4	32.1	5.5
Swordfish	0.54	6.6	2.2	0	46.2	5.4
Tilapia (white fish)	0.58	7.4	0.8	0	36.8	5.8
Trout (farmed)	0.57	6.7	2.1	0	45.7	5.7
Trout (Rainbow, wild)	0.53	6.5	1.7	0	41.3	5.3
Tuna, Bluefin (cooked)	0.67	8.5	1.8	0	50.2	6.7
Tuna, (canned, light in water)	0.43	5.5	0.3	0	24.7	4.3

LEUCINE FACTOR PREFERRED FOODS

FOOD (1-OUNCE SERVING)	LEUCINE (GRAMS)	PROTEIN (GRAMS)	FAT (GRAMS)	CARBS (GRAMS)	CALORIES	LFPs
Tuna (white, canned)	0.54	6.7	0.8	0	34	5.4
Tuna, Yellowfin (cooked)	0.64	8.3	0.2	0	35	6.4
POULTRY (1-OUNCE SERVING)						
Chicken Breast (grilled)	0.72	8.7	0.9	0	42.9	7.2
Egg (1 extra-large egg = 2 oz)	0.33	3.5	2.7	0	38.3	3.3
Egg White (1 extra-large egg white = 1 oz)	0.29	3.1	0	0	12.4	2.9
Egg Yolk (1 extra-large egg yolk = 1 oz)	0.39	4.5	7.5	1	89.5	3.9
Turkey Breast (whole or ground, 97%)	0.53	8.5	0.6	0	39.4	5.3
Turkey (ground, 85%)	0.39	4.8	3.6	0	51.6	3.9
Turkey (ground, lean, 93%)	0.44	5.3	2.4	0	42.8	4.4
DAIRY (1-OUNCE SERVING)						
Colby/ Cheddar (low fat)	0.61	6.9	2	0.5	47.6	6.1
Cottage Cheese (1% fat)	0.36	3.5	0.3	0.8	19.9	3.6
Cottage Cheese (2% fat)	0.3	3	0.6	1.3	22.6	3
Greek Yogurt (0% fat)	0.21	3	0	1.2	16.8	2.1

LEUCINE FACTOR PREFERRED FOODS

FOOD (1-OUNCE SERVING)	LEUCINE (GRAMS)	PROTEIN (GRAMS)	FAT (GRAMS)	CARBS (GRAMS)	CALORIES	LFPs
Gruyere	0.88	8.5	9.2	0.1	117.2	8.8
Milk (2%)	0.1	1.1	0.6	1.6	16.2	1
Milk (Skim)	0.11	1.1	0.1	1.6	11.7	1.1
Mozzarella (low moisture, part-skim)	0.67	6.7	5.6	2.3	86.4	6.7
Parmesan (dry-grated, reduced fat)	0.85	5.7	5.7	0.4	75.7	8.5
Provolone (reduced fat)	0.65	7	5	1	77	6.5
Ricotta (part skim)	0.35	3.2	2.2	1.5	38.6	3.5
Romano Cheese	0.87	9	7.6	1	108.4	8.7
Swiss (low fat)	0.84	7.2	1.4	1.2	46.2	8.4
VEGETARIAN PROTEINS (1-OUNCE SERVING)						
Edamame (frozen, cooked)	0.21	3.7	1.9	3.1	44.3	2.1
Tofu (raw, firm, CaSO4)	0.34	4.5	2.5	1.2	45.3	3.4
FATS (1-OUNCE SERVING)						
Almonds	0.41	6	14.8	6	181.2	4.1
Avocado	0.04	0.6	4.4	2.4	51.6	0.4
Cashews	0.36	4.3	13.1	9.3	172.3	3.6
Flaxseed Oil	0	0	28.4	0	255.6	0
Macadamia Nut Oil	0	0	27.6	0	248.4	0
Macadamia Nuts	0.17	2.2	21.5	3.9	217.9	1.7
Olive Oil	0	0	27	0	243	0
Peanuts	0.44	7.3	14	4.6	173.6	4.4

LEUCINE FACTOR PREFERRED FOODS

FOOD (1-OUNCE SERVING)	LEUCINE (GRAMS)	PROTEIN (GRAMS)	FAT (GRAMS)	CARBS (GRAMS)	CALORIES	LFPs
Pecans	0.175	2.7	21.1	3.8	215.9	1.75
Pistachios	0.45	6.1	13	7.8	172.6	4.5
Walnuts (black)	0.48	6.8	16.7	2.8	188.7	4.8
Walnuts (English)	0.33	4.3	18.5	3.9	199.3	3.3
VEGGIES/FREE FOODS (1-OUNCE SERVING)						
Alfalfa Sprouts	0.08	1.1	0.2	1.1	10.6	0.8
Asparagus	0.04	0.6	0	1.1	6.8	0.4
Broccoli	0.04	0.8	0	1.9	10.8	0.4
Brussels Sprouts	0.04	1	0	2.5	14	0.4
Cauliflower	0.03	0.8	0	1.8	10.4	0.3
Green Beans	0.032	0.5	0	2	10	0.32
Kale	0.05	0.9	0.2	2.8	16.6	0.5
Peas (green)	0.09	1.5	0	4	22	0.9
Peas (sweet)	0.01	0.9	0	2	11.6	0.1
Romaine Lettuce	0.02	0.3	0	0.9	4.8	0.2
Seaweed	0.02	0.5	0.2	2.7	14.6	0.2
Spinach	0.06	0.8	0.1	1	8.1	0.6
Zucchini	0.02	0.3	0	1	5.2	0.2
CARBOHYDRATES (RAW AND DRY) (1-OUNCE SERVING)						
Beets	0.02	0.5	0	2.7	12.8	0.2
Black Beans	0.2	2.5	0.2	6.7	38.6	2
Brown Rice, Raw	0.06	2.1	0.8	21.6	102	0.6
Butternut Squash	0.02	0.3	0	3.3	14.4	0.2
Carrots	0.01	0.3	0	2.7	12	0.1

LEUCINE FACTOR PREFERRED FOODS

FOOD (1-OUNCE SERVING)	LEUCINE (GRAMS)	PROTEIN (GRAMS)	FAT (GRAMS)	CARBS (GRAMS)	CALORIES	LFPs
Couscous	0.07	3.6	0.2	22	104.2	0.7
Ezekiel Bread	0.2	3.3	0.4	12.5	67	2
Kidney Beans	0.21	2.5	0.1	6.5	36.9	2.1
Lentil Beans	0.19	2.6	0.1	5.7	34.1	1.9
Lima Beans	0.19	2.3	0.1	6.6	36.5	1.9
Navy Beans	0.2	2.3	0.2	7.4	40.6	2
Oatmeal	0.36	3.7	1.8	19.2	107.8	3.6
Pinto Beans	0.22	2.6	0.2	7.4	41.8	2.2
Quinoa	0.074	4	1.7	18.2	104.1	0.74
Red Potato	0.03	0.7	0	4.5	20.8	0.3
Soybean	0.25	3.5	1.8	3.1	42.6	2.5
Spelt	0.3	4.1	0.7	19.9	102.3	3
Split Peas	0.17	2.4	0.1	6	34.5	1.7
Sweet Potato	0.03	0.6	0	5.9	26	0.3
White Beans	0.22	2.8	0	7.1	39.6	2.2
White Rice	0.02	2	0.2	22.7	103	0.2
White/Russet Potato	0.03	0.7	0	6	26.8	0.3
Whole Wheat Pasta	0.2	4.1	0.4	21.3	105.2	2
Wild Rice	0.08	4.2	0.3	21.2	104.3	0.8
Yams	0.03	0.4	0	7.8	32.8	0.3

LEUCINE FACTOR PREFERRED FOODS

FOOD (1-OUNCE SERVING)	LEUCINE (GRAMS)	PROTEIN (GRAMS)	FAT (GRAMS)	CARBS (GRAMS)	CALORIES	LFPs
FRUITS (FRESH AND DRIED) (1-OUNCE SERVING)						
Apple	0	0	0	3.9	15.6	0
Apricots (dried)	0	0	0	18.4	73.6	0
Bananas (unripe)	0	0	0	6.5	26	0
Blueberries	0	0	0	4.1	16.4	0
Cherries	0	0	0	4.5	18	0
Elderberries	0	0	0	5.2	20.8	0
Grapefruit	0	0	0	2.3	9.2	0
Grapes (red)	0	0	0	5.1	20.4	0
Guava	0	0	0	4.1	16.4	0
Kiwi	0	0	0	4.2	16.8	0
Mangos	0	0	0	4.4	17.6	0
Oranges	0	0	0	3.3	13.2	0
Papayas	0	0	0	2.8	11.2	0
Pear	0	0	0	4.4	17.6	0
Pineapple	0	0	0	3.7	14.8	0
Prunes	0	0	0	16	64	0
Raisins	0	0	0	22.4	89.6	0
Raspberries	0	0	0	3.4	13.6	0
Strawberries	0	0	0	2.2	8.8	0
Tomatoes	0	0	0	1.1	4.4	0
SUPPLEMENTAL PROTEINS (1-GRAM SERVING)						
Casein	0.088					
Egg Protein Isolate	0.074					
Hemp Protein	0.024					
Soy Isolate	0.067					
Soy Protein	0.046					

LEUCINE FACTOR PREFERRED FOODS

FOOD (1-OUNCE SERVING)	LEUCINE (GRAMS)	PROTEIN (GRAMS)	FAT (GRAMS)	CARBS (GRAMS)	CALORIES	LFPs
Whey Protein Concentrate	0.100					
Whey Protein Isolate	0.110					
STORE SUPPLEMENTS (MEASURED IN SERVING SIZE)						
AboutTime Pancake Mix (1 serving)	2	21	9	30	290	20
AboutTime ProHydrate RTD	2	20	0	3	95	20
AboutTime Whey Protein (1 scoop)	2.5	25	0	1	100	25
GNC BCAA Chew (2 chews)	1.5	2.25	0	7	35	15
GNC Lean Bars (1 bar)	1.2	15	7	22	180	12
GNC Leucine Chew (1 chew)	1.5	1	0.25	2	15	15
GNC PureEdge Vegan (2 scoops)	2	20	2	13	140	20
GNC Total Lean Shake Mix (2 scoops)	2.3	25	3	17	200	23
GNC Total Lean Shake RTD (1 bottle)	2	25	0	6	170	20
GNC Wheybolic 60 Original (1 scoop)	4.56	20	0	2	90	45.6

REFERENCES

Abedini, M., E. Falahi, and S. Roosta. "Dairy Product Consumption and the Metabolic Syndrome." *Diabetology & Metabolic Syndrome* 9, no. 1 (January–March 2015): 34–37.

American Geriatrics Society Workgroup on Vitamin D Supplementation for Older Adults. "Recommendations Abstracted from the American Geriatrics Society Consensus Statement on Vitamin D for Prevention of Falls and Their Consequences." *Journal of the American Geriatrics Society* 62, no. 1 (January 2014): 147–52.

Anderson, Harvey G. and S. E. Moore. "Dietary Proteins in the Regulation of Food Intake and Body Weight in Humans." *Journal of Nutrition* 134, no. 4 (April 2004): 974S–979S.

Anderson, Harvey G., Sandy N. Tecimer, Deepa Shah, and Tasleem A. Zafar. "Protein Source, Quantity, and Time of Consumption Determine the Effect of Proteins on Short-Term Food Intake in Young Men." *Journal of Nutrition* 134, no. 11 (November 1, 2004): 3011–15.

Benton, David and Rachel Donohoe. "The Influence of Creatine Supplementation on the Cognitive Functioning of Vegetarians and Omnivores." *Journal of Nutrition* 105, no. 7 (April 2011): 1100–5.

Burke, Louise M. "Caffeine and Sports Performance." *Applied Physiology, Nutrition, and Metabolism* 33, no. 6 (December 2008): 1319–34.

Burks, Tyesha N., Eva Andres-Mateos, Ruth Marx, Rebeca Mejias, Christel Van Erp, Jessica L. Simmers, Jeremy D. Walston,

Christopher W. Ward, and Ronald D. Cohn. "Losartan Restores Skeletal Muscle Remodeling and Protects Against Disuse Atrophy in Sarcopenia." *Science Translational Medicine* 3, no. 82 (Mary 11, 2011): 82ra37.

Committee on Military Nutrition Research, Food and Nutrition Board. *Caffeine for the Sustainment of Mental Task Performance: Formulations for Military Operations.* Washington, DC: National Academies Press, 2001.

Cooper, Robert, Fernando Naclerio, Judith Allgrove, and Alfonso Jimenez. "Creatine Supplementation with Specific View to Exercise/Sports Performance: An Update." *Journal of the International Society of Sports Nutrition* 9, no. 1 (July 20, 2012): 33.

Davis, J. K. and J. Matt Green. "Caffeine and Anaerobic Performance: Ergogenic Value and Mechanisms of Action." *Sports Med* 39, no. 10 (2009): 813–32.

Dugan, Christine E. and Maria Luz Fernandez. "Effects of Dairy on Metabolic Syndrome Parameters: A Review." *Yale Journal of Biology Medicine* 87, no. 2 (June 2014): 135–47.

Judge, J., S. Birge, F. Gloth 3rd, R. P. Heaney, B. W. Hollis, A. Kenny, D. P. Kiel, D. Saliba, D.L. Schneider, R. Vieth. Recommendations abstracted from the American Geriatrics Society Consensus Statement on vitamin D for Prevention of Falls and Their Consequences. *J Am Geriatr Soc.* 2014 Jan;62(1):147-52.

Kent, K. D., W. J. Harper, and J. A. Bomser. "Effect of Whey Protein Isolate on Intracellular Glutathione and Oxidant-Induced Cell Death in Human Prostate Epithelial Cells." *Toxicology in Vitro* 17, no. 1 (February 2003): 27–33.

Koopman, René, Milou Beelen, Trent Stellingwerff, Bart Pennings, Wim H. M. Saris, Arie K. Kies, Harm Kuipers, and Luc J. C. van Loon. "Coingestion of Carbohydrate with Protein Does Not Further

Augment Postexercise Muscle Protein Synthesis." *American Journal of Physiology: Endocrinology and Metabolism* 293, no. 3 (July 3, 2007): E833–42.

Leenders, Marika and Luc J. C. van Loon. "Leucine as a Pharmaconutrient to Prevent and Treat Sarcopenia and Type 2 Diabetes." *Nutrition Reviews* 69, no. 11 (November 2011): 675–689.

Luhovyy, Bohdan L., Tina Akhavan, and Harvey G. Anderson. "Whey Proteins in the Regulation of Food Intake and Satiety." *Journal of the American College of Nutrition* 26, no. 6 (December 2007): 704S–12S.

Mamerow, Madonna M., Joni A. Mettler, Kirk L. English, Shanon L. Casperson, Emily Arentson-Lantz, Melinda Sheffield-Moore, Donald K. Layman, and Douglas Paddon-Jones. "Dietary Protein Distribution Positively Influences 24-H Muscle Protein Synthesis in Healthy Adults." *Journal of Nutrition* 144, no. 6 (June 1, 2014): 876–80.

Martone, Anna M., Fabrizia Lattanzio, Angela M. Abbatecola, Demenico La Carpia, Matteo Tosato, and Emanuele Marzetti. "Treating Sarcopenia in Older and Oldest Old." *Current Pharmaceutical Design* 21, no. 13 (January 2015): 1715–22.

Mobley, Christopher B., Carlton D. Fox, Brian S. Ferguson, Rajesh H. Amin, Vincent J. Dalbo, Shawn Baier, John A. Rathmacher, Jacob M. Wilson, and Michael D. Roberts. "L-Leucine, Beta-Hydroxy-Beta-Methylbutyric Acid (HMB), and Creatine Monohydrate Prevent Myostatin-Induced Akirin-1/Mighty mRNA Down-Regulation and Myotube Atrophy." *Journal of the International Society of Sports Nutrition* 11 (August 13, 2014): 38.

Motl, Robert W., Patrick J. O'Connor, Leslie Tubandt, Tim Puetz, and Matthew R. Ely. "Effect of Caffeine on Leg Muscle Pain During Cycling Exercise among Females." *Medicine & Science in Sports & Exercise* 38, no. 3 (March 2006): 598–604.

Nissen, S., R. Sharp, M. Ray, J. A. Rathmacher, D. Rice, J. C. Fuller Jr., A. S. Connelly, and N. Abumrad. "Effect of Leucine Metabolite Beta-Hydroxy-Beta-Methylbutyrate on Muscle Metabolism during Resistance-Exercise Training." *Journal of Applied Physiology* 81, no. 5 (November 1, 1996): 2095–104.

Norton, Layne E., Gabriel J. Wilson, Donald K. Layman, Christopher J. Moulton, and Peter J. Garlick. "Leucine Content of Dietary Proteins is a Determinant of Postprandial Skeletal Muscle Protein Synthesis in Adult Rats." *Nutrition & Metabolism* 9, no. 1 (July 20, 2012): 67.

Oike, Hideaki, Katsutaka Oishi, and Masuko Kobori. "Nutrients, Clock Genes, and Chrononutrition." *Current Nutrition Reports* 3, no. 3 (April 27, 2014): 204–12.

Pal, S. and S. Radavelli-Bagatini. "The Effects of Whey Protein on Cardiometabolic Risk Factors." *Obesity Reviews* 14, no. 4 (April 2013): 324–43.

Pasiakos, Stefan M., Holly L. McClung, James P. McClung, Lee M. Margolis, Nancy E. Anderson, Gregory J. Cloutier, Matthew A. Pikosky, Jennifer C. Rood, Roger A. Fielding, and Andrew J. Young. "Leucine-Enriched Essential Amino Acid Supplementation during Moderate Steady State Exercise Enhances Postexercise Muscle Protein Synthesis." *American Journal of Clinical Nutrition* 94, no. 3 (September 2011): 809–18.

Petersen, Brent L., Loren S. Ward, Eric D. Bastian, Alexandra L. Jenkins, Janice Campbell, and Vladimir Vuksan. "A Whey Protein Supplement Decreases Post-Prandial Glycemia." *Nutrition Journal* 8, no. 47 (October 16, 2009). Accessed 2015. doi: 10.1186/1475-2891-8-47.

Pihlanto-Leppälä, Anne, Päivi Koskinen, Kati Piilola, Tuomo Tupasela, and Hannu Korhonen. "Angiotensin I-Converting Enzyme Inhibitory Properties of Whey Protein Digests:

Concentration and Characterization of Active Peptides." *Journal of Dairy Research* 67, no. 1 (February 2000): 53–64.

Salles, Jérôme, Audrey Chanet, Christophe Giraudet, Véronique Patrac, Philippe Pierre, and Marion Jourdan. "1,25(OH)2-Vitamin D3 Enhances the Stimulating Effect of Leucine and Insulin on Protein Synthesis Rate through Akt/PKB and mTOR Mediated Pathways in Murine C2C12 Skeletal Myotubes." *Molecular Nutrition & Food Research* 57, no. 12 (December 2013): 2137–46.

Sepkowitz, Kent A. "Energy Drinks and Caffeine-Related Adverse Effects." *Journal of the American Medical Association* 309, no. 3 (January 16, 2013): 243–44.

Speakman, John R., Elżbieta Król, and Maria S. Johnson. "The Functional Significance of Individual Variation in Basal Metabolic Rate." *Physiological and Biochemical Zoology* 77, no. 6 (November/December 2004): 900–915.

Stanhope, Kimber L., Jean Marc Schwarz, Nancy L. Keim, Steven C. Griffen, Andrew A. Bremer, James L. Graham, Bonnie Hatcher, Chad L. Cox, Artem Dyachenko, Wei Zhang, John P. McGahan, Anthony Seibert, Ronald M. Krauss, Sally Chiu, Ernst J. Schaefer, Masumi Ai, Seiko Otokozawa, Katsuyuki Nakajima, Takamitsu Nakano, Carine Beysen, Marc K. Hellerstein, Lars Berglund, and Peter J. Havel. "Consuming Fructose-Sweetened, Not Glucose-Sweetened, Beverages Increases Visceral Adiposity and Lipids and Decreases Insulin Sensitivity in Overweight/Obese Humans." *Journal of Clinical Investigation* 119, no. 5 (April 20, 2009): 1322–34.

Tang, Jason E., Daniel R. Moore, Gregory W. Kujbida, Mark A. Tarnopolsky, and Stuart M. Phillips. "Ingestion of Whey Hydrolysate, Casein, or Soy Protein Isolate: Effects on Mixed Muscle Protein Synthesis at Rest and Following Resistance Exercise in Young Men." *Journal of Applied Physiology* 107, no. 3 (September 1, 2009): 987–92.

Volpi, Elena, Hisamine Kobayashi, Melinda Sheffield-Moore, Bettina Mittendorfer, and Robert R. Wolfe. "Essential Amino Acids Are Primarily Responsible for the Amino Acid Stimulation of Muscle Protein Anabolism in Healthy Elderly Adults." *American Journal of Clinical Nutrition* 78, no. 2 (August 2003): 250–8.

Wilson, Jacob M., Peter J. Fitschen, Bill Campbell, Gabriel J. Wilson, Nelo Zanchi, Lem Taylor, Colin Wilborn, Douglas S. Kalman, Jeffrey R. Stout, Jay R. Hoffman, Tim N. Ziegenfuss, Hector L. Lopez, Richard B. Kreider, Abbie E. Smith-Ryan, and Jose Antonio. "International Society of Sports Nutrition Position Stand: Beta-Hydroxy-Beta-Methylbutyrate (HMB)." *Journal of the International Society of Sports Nutrition* 10, no. 1 (February 2, 2013): 6.

Wyon, Matthew A., Yiannis Koutedakis, Roger Wolman, Alan M. Nevill, and Nick Allen. "The Influence of Winter Vitamin D Supplementation on Muscle Function and Injury Occurrence in Elite Ballet Dancers: a Controlled Study." *Journal of Science and Medicine in Sport* 17, no. 1 (April 25, 2013): 8–12.

Zemel, Michael B. "Mechanisms of Dairy Modulation of Adiposity." *Journal of Nutrition* 133, no. 1 (January 1, 2003): 252S–256S.

Zhang, Yiying, Kaiying Guo, Robert E. LeBlanc, Daniella Loh, Gary J. Schwartz, and Yi-Hao Yu. "Increasing Dietary Leucine Intake Reduces Diet-Induced Obesity and Improves Glucose and Cholesterol Metabolism in Mice via Multimechanisms." *Diabetes* 56, no. 6 (March 14, 2007): 1647–54.

Zioudrou, Christine, Richard A. Streaty, and Werner A. Klee. "Opioid Peptides Derived from Food Proteins: The Exorphins." *Journal of Biological Chemistry* 254, no. 7 (April 10, 1979): 2446–9.

INDEX

ACKNOWLEDGMENTS

I would like to thank the following individuals and organizations for their continued support:

- Jim Manion of the National Physique Committee and the International Federation for Bodybuilding for his guidance, friendship, and constant support.

- John Paul and the Allegheny Health Network for supporting my patients and their needs.

- General Nutrition Centers and the GNC medical advisory board for their motivation and desire to improve human health and nutrition.

- Steve Blechman and Advanced Research Media for giving me a place to share my knowledge with the world of bodybuilding and fitness.

- Chef Donato Coluccio for his culinary expertise, companionship, and recipes shared in this book.

- The Ulysses Press editorial team for their faith in my writing.

- My wife, family, and friends, who put up with my need to be on the move to make the world a better place. #BetterThanYesterdaysSelf

ABOUT THE AUTHOR

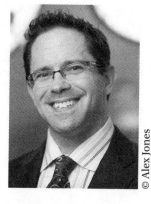

© Alex Jones

Dr. Victor Prisk is a board-certified orthopedic surgeon, national champion bodybuilder, All-American gymnast, and professional swing dancer. He is a popular fitness expert in print, digital, and broadcast media. As a member of the General Nutrition Centers (GNC) medical advisory board, he has contributed to product development, instructional videos, blogs, and print media. Previously, he served as a physician and athlete spokesman for one of the largest supplement companies in the world, Muscletech, of Iovate Health Sciences.

An avid writer, Dr. Prisk serves on the editorial board of Steve Blechman's Advanced Research Media with columns in *Muscular Development Magazine, Fitness Rx for Men,* and *Fitness Rx for Women.* He authors columns and contributes content to *Muscle and Fitness, Flex, Wellbella,* and *Muscle* and *Body* magazines. He has also written articles translated into many languages and published in international magazines including *Physique Magazine* in Dubai and *Sport en Fitness Magazine* in the Netherlands.

Dr. Prisk is active in social media marketing campaigns as an elite content contributor for the increasingly popular company FitFluential.com and HealthHaven app. He is also active on social media including Instagram, Facebook, Twitter, and Periscope. He has developed numerous nutritional formulas with GNC and SDC Nutrition, including the "Factor Series" led by The OrthoFactor AM/PM Mobility Formula. You can find Dr. Prisk @DrVictorPrisk on IG, @VictorPrisk on Twitter, and online at LeucineFactor.com.